Accidental
Psychiatrist

Accidental Psychiatrist

THE HEALING POWER OF COMPASSION

Bob Kamath M.D.

K. P. S. "Bob" Kamath, address: 2029 Andrew Drive, Cape Girardeau, MO
63701, U.S.A. pkamath001@gmail.com
Author's other works: Servants, Not Masters (1986), Is Your Balloon About To
Pop? (2007), The Untold Story of the Bhagavad Gita (2013), Ashoka's Song in
the Bhagavad Gita (2016).

ISBN: 154064037X
ISBN 13: 9781540640376

Contents

Dedication

I dedicate this book to all my patients who taught me all that I know about psychiatry. I am ever grateful to them for their kindness and support throughout my career in psychiatry.

Author to Reader

IN THIS BOOK I HOPE to reveal to readers the healing power of compassion, while giving them a glimpse into my life as a psychiatrist in America. Writing this book has been a difficult endeavor, as I had to relive some painful emotions related to long-forgotten traumatic events.

When I was in practice, my patients often told me that I had the reputation for telling it as it is. I am not about to change that essential element of my persona.

Over the past five decades compassion, an essential element of medical practice, seems to have gradually diminished. Increasingly the noble medical profession has tended to become a business transaction.

Between 1975 and 1984, my little boy underwent twenty-six surgical procedures for the treatment of fracture of femur and surgical complications due to a doctor's negligence. Four of these were major surgeries requiring blood transfusion.

Of the five orthopedic surgeons who operated on my boy in five reputable hospitals in St. Louis, Boston and New York, only one of them met with us briefly before surgery, and none of them had anything to do with us afterwards. They were not any different from auto mechanics that serviced my cars. None said a kind word; none gave us any hope, or follow-up care. Once they did their "job," they were done with us. They could not have cared less about the suffering of my little boy or our parental anguish. None of them had any 'blood in the eye,' as my heartbroken wife expressed it in tears while waiting for long hours in the waiting rooms. All that mattered to them was that they got the huge fee they charged us. And they all knew that I was a physician.

In 1984, a "reputable doctor" in New York City, about whose orthopedic skill Time Magazine wrote a full-page article, demanded $14,000 in advance before making an appointment. I paid him, but I never met him either before or after the three-hour long surgery. I would not have believed the callousness of this famous doctor had I not been at the receiving end of it.

I am sure there are thousands of compassionate and caring doctors in America. However, during the course of my long psychiatric practice, I lost count of patients who told me horror stories of their contacts with doctors and hospitals. They never shared their anguish with their doctors for fear of hurting them.

And I have lost count of people I treated for *medical trauma,* a serious emotional disorder resulting from callous medical treatment and complications thereof by compassionless doctors and other medical staff. Complacent medical profession is yet to recognize this doctor-induced disorder as real, and accept responsibility for it.

Over the past four decades psychiatry has increasingly become "medicalized," and exclusive drug treatment of emotional disorders has become 'The State of the Art.' Empathic exploration of underlying emotional issues (psychodynamics) seems to have fallen by the wayside, mainly because it is difficult to practice, time consuming for the untrained, and there is not much profit in it. Drug-oriented cookbook remedy has replaced it because it is far easier and far more lucrative. Now drug companies have assumed the responsibility of "educating" psychiatrists as well as the general public about the virtues of symptomatic drug treatment of emotional disorders. Symptomatic treatment has replaced cure. The nexus of drug companies and psychiatric community has become the proverbial elephant in the room. Everyone is pretending not to notice it.

No doubt, psychiatric drugs have an important role to play in the treatment of emotional and mental disorders. However, exclusive drug treatment, i.e. without concurrent psychotherapy and education, is fraught with serious long-term consequences to patients' physical as well as mental health. Complacent psychiatric profession is yet to accept its role in creating the so-called *refractory* or *drug-resistant* cases.

In some of the chapters I have quoted verbatim a few unsolicited letters I received from my ex-patients, only as evidence to the healing power of compassion for their suffering, helpfulness in alleviating it and education to prevent it in the future.

Dr. Bob Kamath   January 2017

Part One

The Psychiatric Practice

CHAPTER 1

Physician, Heal Thyself

Luke 4:23: And he said unto them, Ye will surely say unto
me this proverb, Physician, heal thyself: whatsoever we have
heard done in Capernaum, do also here in thy country.

WHEN IN JULY 1970 I joined Elmhurst General Hospital in New
York City as an 'Rotating Intern,' I had just graduated from a
medical school in India. My plan was to receive three years of
training as Resident in Internal Medicine beginning in 1971,
followed by two years of fellowship in Cardiology beginning in
1974. The medical training program in this hospital was affiliated with the famous Mount Sinai Hospital of New York City.

Immediately after joining the hospital, however, I was
shocked to note that the medical treatment offered to seriously
ill patients in this hospital was almost totally devoid of compassion for their suffering. I spent the first two months in the emergency room where patients with serious medical problems were
brought, such as heart attacks, strokes, diabetic coma, asthmatic

attacks, epilepsy, gunshot wounds, knife wounds, broken bones, head injuries, overdoses, pneumonia, pulmonary embolism, and just about every malady that offered wonderful opportunity for me to learn American medicine. Instead, due to total absence of any teaching, my so-called *medical training* consisted of drawing blood, starting I.V. drips, pushing patients to X-ray rooms, and doing other menial tasks, which were normally done by orderlies, nurses and laboratory technicians. I learned absolutely nothing.

This was also the situation when I rotated through other departments. There was little teaching, and working 36 hours in a stretch left me feeling exhausted, and with little time for my private life, or to read medical journals. Today these dehumanizing practices could pass for human trafficking. It dawned on me that the affiliation of this hospital with Mount Sinai Hospital of New York City was merely a bait to attract cheap medical labor to this godforsaken city hospital.

What was even more alarming to me was that this 'medical training program' forced me to become part of impersonal medical system geared primarily to enhance revenue for the hospital. Being the lowest person on this medical totem pole, I was the designated person to deliver the compassionless patient care, and I had neither a say about its quality nor the right to refuse to do it.

In a sense what I was experiencing was the clash between highly *personalized* Indian medical culture of which I was a part, and highly *impersonal* American medical culture, which I had now become a part of. To me medical treatment was more an *art of healing people;* to the American doctors that I met there, it was mostly a *science of treating disorders.* To me compassion for patients' suffering was *central* to the healing process. To the American doctors, however, offering scientifically appropriate treatment was *essential* for the patients' recovery. Ideally these two diverse approaches should be inseparably combined in all medical treatments. But I did not have the needed training or power to accomplish this feat, as I had just arrived from a country half way across the globe. I felt trapped in this grossly alien system, as I had no money to buy the return ticket to India, and I could not break the contract I had signed to serve the hospital for one year.

The head-spinning events that I witnessed in this hospital over the next six months forced me to give up the pursuit of the *science* of treating damaged hearts, and pursue the *art* of mending broken hearts. And the first broken heart I had to mend was my own. Psychiatry perfectly suited my innate temperament: compassion for others' suffering and irresistible compulsion to help those in dire distress. Thus I became a psychiatrist by sheer accident, and very likely to heal myself from my one-year long traumatic experiences in the hospital as well as in New York City.

In Chapters 8 and 9, I have described my unending ordeals with Elmhurst General Hospital, beginning with my heartbreaking interaction with its utterly callous Chief Administrator within 30 minutes of landing in New York. I narrowly missed spending my first night on a sidewalk of New York City, like so many homeless people did those days.

Establishing private practice: After completing 3-year long so-called training in psychiatry in Connecticut in 1974, I worked successively as *inpatient* psychiatrist in three psychiatric hospitals before opening my primarily *outpatient* private practice in 1982 in Cape Girardeau, Missouri, a small town in the Heartland of America. However, all the experience I had gained treating seriously ill *dysfunctional inpatients* with drugs and supportive therapy was of little help to me in treating *functioning outpatients* suffering from relatively milder psychiatric ailments rooted in complex 'traumatic emotional issues.' They were farmers, housewives, teachers, professors, doctors, nurses, lawyers, administrators, laborers, and the like. They complained of depression, suicidal impulses, anxiety, panic attacks, fainting spells, headache attacks, pain somewhere in the body, impotence, and many other symptoms for which their personal physicians and various specialists had found no physical basis. Suspecting a psychological basis for their symptoms, their doctors referred them to me.

Traumatic emotional issues: In a case, such as a Viet Nam veteran suffering from posttraumatic stress disorder (PTSD), it was quite obvious to the patient as well as me what brought on his disorder: his wartime traumatic experience. He suffered from 'flashbacks' every time a sound, sight, taste, touch or smell reminded him of his trauma on the battlefield. The problem in treating run-of-the-mill patients was that they were simply *not aware* of their past and present traumatic experiences.

For example, a man suffering from severe panic attacks would say, "I have no stress at all in my life. I had no childhood traumas at all. I had a wonderful childhood." Yet, I knew that in a lesser sense, he was also a victim of posttraumatic stress disorder. In order to help this miserable man, I must play the *mind detective,* discover his hidden 'traumatic emotional issues,' and help him to make the connection between them and his panic disorder.

In the interview, this young man reveals that his panic attack started the day after he celebrated the birthday of his four-year old boy. He has no memory of the tragic event of his father's death in a car accident when he was four years old. The challenge for me is to elicit this information from this young man and help him to make sense of his panic attacks in the light of his father's tragic death over 25 years ago.

Psychodynamics: Psychiatrists refer to the 'traumatic emotional issues' underlying emotional disorders by a high-sounding term: *psychodynamics.* This psychiatric term simply means *'understanding patients' disorder in the light of their thoughts, emotions and behaviors rooted in their past traumatic experiences.'*

To a greater or lesser degree we are all products of our past traumatic experiences such as bereavement, divorce, parental conflict, breakup of family, abandonment, betrayal, financial ruin, emotional, physical and sexual abuse, alcoholism of parents, injustice, and other tragedies of life. These traumatic experiences stamp lasting impressions on our mind and determine the entire course of our lives. Most of them leave serious 'emotional scars.' In a sense, most of us are 'damaged goods,' and yet we managed to survive and move on with our lives. Our past is who we are today.

In some people these traumatic experiences ultimately result in *emotional disorders*, such as depression, bipolar disorder, panic disorder, obsessive-compulsive disorder, social phobia, pain disorder, etc.

In some others they result in *disorders of personality*, such as paranoid personality, obsessive-compulsive personality, antisocial personality, narcissistic personality, etc. These people are like miniature bonsai trees, which are shaped by chronic deprivation of nutrients, frequent pruning, twisting of branches by wires and by weights. Just as bonsai trees cannot be changed into normal trees, it is almost impossible to change the innate character of these people.

In still others the past traumatic experience manifest as a distinct, well established *pattern of behavior* such as showing off one's wealth, making money by hook or by crook, competing with others, winning at any cost, and many other such persistent behaviors.

In many others they stimulate incredible creativity in art, science, politics, business, military, and many other fields of human endeavors.

A case study: Let me give the reader an example of how a severely traumatic experience I had as a boy left lasting emotional scars in my mind and created a *pattern of behavior* I displayed all my life including during my psychiatric practice:

When I was 6 years old, two neighborhood kids, each about twice my size, bullied me mercilessly. When I returned home from school, often they stood at the entrance of the four-story apartment building where I lived, and chased me and kicked my butt. I often stood scared on the sidewalk, looked up at the fourth floor apartment where my family lived, and called out my older brother to rescue me, and occasionally he did. Every evening I dreaded coming home from school. Even at that tender age, I continually felt humiliated and terribly helpless. This bullying went on for three years.[1]

When I was 9 years old, my family moved from Mumbai to my father's hometown Karkala, 500 miles to the south. By then I must have decided never to let anyone bully me again, as evidenced by the fact that I lost all fear of bullies. Because I was seen as a city boy, several country boys began to bully me. With reckless disregard for my safety I got into fights with them. On one occasion, I tore off a bully's shirt, and he had to go home bare-chested in shame. Soon bullies in my class began to fear me and there was no more bullying.

By the time I joined high school, 'zero tolerance for bullies' became my mantra. To deal with bullying hoodlums in my class, I went to the local gymnasium and took up bodybuilding. When these hoodlums came to know that I could lift over my head a barbell weighing greater than my own body weight, and when they witnessed me doing 20 pull-ups nonstop, they all quit bullying and became my friends. I protected my younger brothers from bullies, and on one occasion even risked being killed by a gang of hoodlums.

This reckless *behavioral pattern* of 'fighting bullies' continued in medical school. On one occasion, for no good reason a bully berated me in front of a large number of people.[2] I walked away from him to avoid a public spectacle. He followed me and

---

1 Bullying is a highly traumatic experience for children. Many bullied children commit suicide unable to cope with it.

2 I call this Wyatt Earp syndrome. Bullies test people who have the reputation for not tolerating bullies. They always think they would win. Wyatt Earp killed all the gunfighters who bullied him. He died of old age.

threatened to "kick your butt." I was determined never to let anyone kick my butt again. I told him that if he ever touched me, he would regret it rest of his life. He called me a coward and touched my chin saying, "What will you do if I touched you, you coward?" That was all I needed to make him remember me the rest of his life. With my fist I hit him on the mouth once so hard that I knocked off several of his front teeth and bloodied his mouth. He flew eight feet away, picked up his teeth from the floor screaming and yelling profanities, and bleeding profusely he ran to the emergency room. I hated to do this, but he left me with no choice. My childhood trauma dictated that I never suffer bullying in silence again. I faced serious consequences due to this incident, but I never regretted what I did.

This pattern of 'zero tolerance for bullies' behavior continued even in my psychiatric practice. Whenever any organization bullied me, I fought back. When the Medical Director of General Medical Insurance of Medicare sent me a threatening letter for no good reason, I drove all the way to St. Louis, confronted him, and told him that I did not need Medicare in my practice, and if he ever threatened me again I would resign from Medicare. He backed off.[3]

I resigned from Medicare in 1998 after the new law permitted doctors to opt-out of Medicare and treat patients as their private clients. Not knowing that I was not with Medicare, an ignorant official of General American told several of my patients, "There is no doctor who is not with Medicare. If your doctor tells you otherwise, he is a fraud. Report him to the Fraud Line." I called

---

3 In 2002, American General Insurance agreed to pay $76 million in fine after the U.S. sued it for fraud.

Medicare immediately and demanded an apology in writing or face a libel lawsuit. Within two days I received an unconditional apology letter from Medicare.

When Proctor and Gamble Company threatened to stop referring their employees to me unless I stopped telling their sick employees that *swing shift* was rather bad for their physical, mental and family health, with total disregard to the consequences I told them, "Go ahead. Make my day!" So P&G forbade their employees from seeing me for treatment. The same thing happened with Southwestern Bell. I lost a lot of income, but I told myself that no company, however powerful, has the right to bully me, and dictate to me what I should or should not tell my patients.

When around 1997 Managed Care became the mantra of the day, and Health Maintenance Organizations (HMO) began to dictate to me what I could do or not do, I resigned from them all, and practiced psychiatry completely independent of them. When HMO executives showed up at my office and tried to dissuade me from resigning, I told them that so long as they tried to dictate my practice, I would not be part of their chicanery. I told them that I would beg in the streets before submitting to their threats. Thus I gave up a great deal of income, and even prepared to shut down my practice. That was the price I had to pay for my liberty and self-respect.[4]

However, I did not have to shut down my practice. My principled stance to do what was best for my patients earned me the

---

4 During the recent presidential election, I was appalled by the fact that neither the 16 Republican presidential candidates nor the two elected Republican leaders had the guts to stand up to Donald Trump when he bullied and berated them. I lost all respect for these cowardly 'leaders.'

reputation in this town as 'the doctor who could not be intimidated or bought.' This instilled in people confidence in my integrity, and a lot of people consulted me as 'out of network doctor,' and I made a very good living from my practice till my retirement at age 65 in 2010. I retired with my head held high.

Blast from the past: There is another aspect to the psychodynamics of childhood or even adulthood. Some people bury painful emotions related to life traumas in their *hidden mind* and move on with life as if nothing ever happened. Burying painful emotions gives people immediate and significant relief from their distress.[5] Over time people forget their old trauma, and move on with their life. Psychiatrists call this phenomenon 'repression.' However, like an unexploded bomb buried ten feet underground, the emotional trauma remains more or less away from one's awareness. A later seemingly insignificant good or bad event could trigger the buried traumatic emotions to suddenly resurface and cause a serious emotional disorder such as major depression, panic disorder, pain syndrome, postpartum depression/psychosis, etc. It is like an accidental strike of a pickaxe triggering the buried bomb to blow up. The best way I can explain this is by using the following model: Imagine a balloon attached to the top of a soda bottle filled with gaseous soda. If we shake the soda bottle vigorously, the gas in the soda would be released, and it would spew up into the inflated balloon and pop it. I call this phenomenon "double whammy" (see picture#16 in Chapter Seven). In Chapter Four I have discussed two such 'blast from the past' cases.

---

5   We refer to this immediate relief from distress by the term 'primary gain.'

Sometimes, however, the resurfacing buried traumatic emotional issues *compel people to act* on them and attempt to resolve them once and for all.[6] We are all familiar with the stories of people who abruptly left their lucrative jobs or businesses and heeded a 'calling' to do something they considered as more meaningful and satisfying.

A case study: Let me give the reader an example of how a buried traumatic emotional issue from my own childhood suddenly resurfaced when I was 30 years old, and how I *helplessly* acted on it to resolve it. To all my family members, including my wife, my parents, my siblings, and in in-laws, my actions were totally irrational. My mother said that taking care of crazy people must have made me also crazy. Only in hindsight was I able to understand the psychodynamic basis of my "irrational" behavior:

Shortly after my birth in 1945, my father launched a commercial bank, which he named after me hoping that I would bring him good luck. By the time I was four years old, however, the bank began to falter due to unexpected changes in the policies of the Reserve Bank of India. Finally the bank went under when I was seven year old. My father must have felt that I brought him bad luck. He treated me harshly for several years during these difficult times in his life. Perhaps sensing his anger and rejection, I cried a lot between the ages of four and seven, and my father often chastised me that there must be huge water tank inside my head.

---

6 'Midlife crisis' is an example of how adults indulge in extramarital affairs to fulfill their unmet needs from childhood to be loved and admired. A small event usually triggers resurfacing of these unmet needs.

Some degree of verbal and physical abuse continued till I was 12 years old. I never saw him behave this way with my siblings.

I grew up feeling that I was somehow responsible for my father's misfortune and that he hated me for it. I got the impression that he thought that I would amount to nothing as an adult. Pervasive feelings of guilt, shame and worthlessness haunted me during my teenage years. To make matter worse, my mother often referred to me as 'the ugly one' among her children, as I was somewhat darker than my siblings. I was ashamed to face a crowd of people. In fact, even going into a crowded restaurant scared me to death. Modern psychiatrists would have diagnosed me as suffering from an anxiety disorder known as social phobia. Gradually these painful emotions went underground and I moved on with my life.

Fast forward to 1975. When my first born boy was one year old, suddenly I began to have irresistible urge to return to India to "do some fundamental work there," though I had no idea what that could be. It was a 'calling' I just could not resist. Every waking moment I thought, 'I've got to go back home and do something worthwhile.' Even in my dreams this theme kept recurring. Fighting injustice in India became an obsession with me. I compulsively read history books on India and studied biography of Mahatma Gandhi for the next four years to prepare myself for my anticipated 'struggle' in India.

Compelled to act on this irresistible obsession, I quit the high-paying job of Medical Director of a Community Mental Health Center (CMHC), sold my house, cars, furniture and all my possessions, and returned to India with my wife and two little children in December 1979. My wife and my poor parents were appalled by my foolish decision. I was so driven by my obsession that I did not care what anyone thought or said.

Back in India, after overcoming many obstacles, I started a grass-roots consumer movement against institutionalized corruption and injustice, and published a newspaper to mobilize public support. I held huge public meetings to raise people's awareness about the problem of corruption and injustice in every Indian bureaucracy. Crowds did not scare me anymore. In fact, I enjoyed addressing huge crowds and meeting hundreds of people. Big shots came to meet me at my home, and offered their cooperation. The movement was so successful that soon it spread to many neighboring districts. There was widespread admiration for the work I did to fight injustice in the society.

In the process of this 18-month long successful struggle with corrupt bureaucracies I liberated myself from the deep-rooted feelings of guilt, shame and worthlessness, and thus redeemed myself. The whole experience was 'therapy' for my childhood traumatic emotional issue. When I returned to America in May 1981, I felt like a completely different person: full of self-confidence and boundless energy. Nothing scared me anymore. It was as if I had just overthrown a ton of weight from my shoulders. I took up the challenging job of Chief of Medical Staff of a large dying State Hospital and succeeded in reviving it within one year.

But my issues with my father still remained to be resolved. After returning to America, I continued to be involved in the consumer rights movement in India. In 1986 I published a definitive guide on this movement titled, 'Servants, Not Masters,' subtitled 'A Guide for Consumer Activists in India.' It was released in a huge public function in my hometown. Leading newspapers of India hailed this book as "the Bible of Consumer Movement in India." It received highly appreciative reviews from a few literary giants. I became a well-known person in the political and bureaucratic circles of State of Karnataka. The local Member of Parliament (M.P.) Oscar Fernandez, an acquaintance from my boyhood days, and an ardent supporter of our movement, worked closely with his friend Prime Minister Rajiv Gandhi, and helped to pass the Consumer Protection Act (1986). The Government of India established over 700 Consumer Courts across the country to address consumer grievances. (Check Google).

In 1988, when I visited India to attend the statewide convention on consumer education that I had sponsored, I met my father. Though he was well known and highly respected in the community by his own right, by then people often referred to him as the father of the man who founded the consumer movement. For the first time in my life I felt that he was proud of me. Just before I left for America, for the first time in my life I hugged him, and he sobbed. I had never seen him shed a tear before.

I had made my peace with him none too soon. For, shortly after that he suffered a massive stroke, which destroyed over one half of his brain, and he was unable to speak and swallow food. A few months before he died, I met him for the last time and videotaped our interaction. I asked him, "Dad, do you know who I am?" He shook his head affirmatively, extended his right hand a little, made a hand gesture, struggled to talk, but only managed to mumble something. My mother, who had learned to understand his gestures and mumbles, interpreted him to me: "He said, 'You are the son who sent money to him from America.'" Yes, I had sent him money every single month without fail ever since I came to America in 1970, and even when one half of his brain had died he remembered my help with gratitude. When he died in 1991, his obituary mentioned, "His second son is Dr. Prabhakar Kamath, the founder of Consumers Forum of Udupi."

In November 2000, the 586-page Commemorative Publication released on the occasion of 200th anniversary of the District of South Canara, titled 'POLI, CANARA 200,' devoted an entire chapter to my work in the field of consumer rights, and declared it as a historical achievement.

Had I not resolved this resurfacing traumatic emotional issue of my childhood before my father's death, I would have certainly suffered from chronic feelings of sadness and discontent in life. No amount of psychotherapy could have helped me. Unfortunately, I had to put my wife and two little boys through hell in the process of liberating myself from my 'demons.' I often consoled my wife Geetha, "Had I not done all this, I would have gone crazy. You wouldn't want to live with a chronically depressed husband, would you? Thank you for standing by me. I will never put you through anything like this again. I promise."

Overthrowing the burdens of my past traumatic emotional issues liberated my intellectual creativity. I wrote several more books: 'Secrets of Stress Management,' 'Is Your Balloon About To Pop?' 'The Untold Story of the Bhagavad Gita,' 'Ashoka's Song in the Bhagavad Gita,' and now 'Accidental Psychiatrist.' In all of these books, I offered readers something entirely original. I have several more books in the making.

This was how I learned to make compost out of garbage life gave me.

Are you all right, doctor? When I established my private practice in 1982, however, it was not easy for me to figure out my patients' psychodynamics. This situation was like a general surgeon having to perform brain surgery. Eliciting psychodynamic information from functioning patients required special interview skills, and making sense of it required a thorough knowledge of how the mind worked. I was so stressed by the sudden switch to the *outpatient setting* that on one occasion a middle-aged man I was interviewing offered me a handful of tissue papers to wipe the profuse sweat pouring down from my forehead, and asked, "Are you all right, doctor?" Luckily, during this early stage of my private practice, my patients did not know that I was sweating because I was struggling to figure out their unique psychodynamics. My medical degree, diploma in psychiatry, and reputation as a psychiatrist fooled them into believing that I must know what I was doing.

However, my own *sufferings* in life had sensitized me to my patients' sufferings, and *motivated me to help* them as best as I could. Now these two qualities became two essential tools in my practice. I listened to my patients empathically and did what I could to promptly alleviate their misery with medication, supportive therapy and common sense advice. What struck me was that my obvious compassion for their sufferings and empathic listening not only healed them but also induced them to give me insight into the psychodynamics I needed to help them. For every sincere empathic statement I made, they rewarded me with an important bit of information I needed to put the jigsaw puzzle of their life together. What surprised me was that they gave me information even before I asked them the question I intended to ask. It was as if there was telepathic communication between us.

They basked in the comfort of talking to someone who understood them perfectly, without judging or criticizing them.

The reader might ask: What was the proof for this assertion? Well, shortly after their recovery, invariably they referred their relatives and friends to me for treatment. When I asked new patients, "Who gave you my name?" invariably they said, "So-and-so that you saw two weeks ago told me 'you must see this guy.'" Thus my practice flourished mostly due to the word-of-mouth referrals by my ex-patients.

In a real sense, it was not by accident that I became a psychiatrist. Nor was it an accident that my psychiatric practice became highly successful. My past traumatic experiences determined what I became and set the tone to how I treated my patients.[7] I am reminded of Jesus' words: Mathew 11:29: "Take my yoke upon you and learn from me, for I am humble and gentle at heart, and you will find rest for your souls."

Learning from my patients: In fact, my real training in eliciting psychodynamics of my patients began only after I started my private practice in 1982. Hundreds upon hundreds of patients taught me what no book or training program could. I heard one statement from just about every patient I listened to: *I just can't take it anymore!* This was the clue that they were at their *emotional breaking point.* Painful emotions such as fear, hurt, anger, sadness, guilt, shame, disappointment, etc. had built up in their mind like

---

7 Behavior of both 'no drama Obama' and 'high drama Trump' is based on their respective childhood traumatic experiences. In the former they gave him self-assurance; and in the latter, they made him insecure, which led to his behavioral pattern of bragging, hyperbole, lying, and berating others, and made him a textbook case of narcissistic personality.

air filling a balloon, and their balloon was about to pop. They did not know how to express these painful feelings and calm themselves down. That is why they needed my help to, well, 'shrink' their balloon. I could readily relate to this state of mind, as I had experienced that feeling several times while growing up in India, not to mention during the first few years of my life in America. All I had to do was to listen to them empathically, and they expressed their pent-up emotions freely and felt better.

A terminally ill patient came to see me week after week for a few weeks before she died. I just listened to her empathically without saying much. What could I say to someone who was dying? She cried her heart out during every session. Before she died she dedicated a poem to me and wrote the following poignant letter:

To you, Dr. Kamath, for so many things.

First, the inspiration to write this. You knew all along, didn't you, that it would be a catharsis for all my <u>pent up emotions?</u>

Secondly, thank you for <u>being there</u> for me, patient and willing to listen —even to find some meaning to my silences.

And finally, thank you for becoming a friend who is still working on putting the pieces of my mind back together. The poem on p. 19, dedicated to you, does not in any way do justice to the help you have given me.

I will always thank the heavens that you were the person I went to see when all was black and scary.
Sincerely,
L. P.

In Chapter Three, we will read two rather dramatic case studies to further illustrate how my compassionate listening helped two patients to express pent-up painful emotions, and mended their broken hearts.

Over the years, as my patients taught me better interviewing skills, and offered more insight into their mind, I developed a model of the mind -a template- which enabled me to figure out the psychodynamics of even very complicated cases within 30 minutes sans sweat. I have explained this model in great detail in Chapter 7. The benefit this model gave me was such that I was able to see a very large number of patients and figure out their psychodynamics very easily in a very short time. We will study psychodynamics of two complicated cases in Chapter 4. Developing the model of mind made my practice become more and more enjoyable. I never thought that there would come a time when every morning I eagerly looked forward to testing my model on new as well as established patients. I realized then that few professions could be as interesting as psychiatry.

Developing the model of the mind helped me in another important way: It gave me insight into my own psychodynamics. It helped me to figure out the bases of my past follies and present behavioral quirks. Insight into my own mind gave me the ability to put things in proper perspective and heal myself. Thus I validated the ancient wisdom, 'Physician, heal thyself' while healing others.

Playing the mind detective: As a psychiatrist I played the mind detective to unravel the psychodynamics of my patients' mind by judicious questioning, empathic listening, intensely observing and applying the power of deduction. For example, if a 'happily married' woman complained of inexplicable headache attacks every night, she might have an issue with her husband. That issue would need to be *gently and indirectly* explored, for, if I asked her directly about her husband, she might say something like, "Oh, he is such a wonderful man. I love him to death." In every case, I had to use the technique of what I call *stealth interview* to break through patient's denial ("everything is wonderful in my life") and blaming others ("my mother-in-law is the cause of all my headaches"). Many patients thought that we were just having a superfluous chat and not a formal psychiatric interview. All the while during this 'tête-à-tête,' I was secretly gathering all the information I needed to know their psychodynamics. At the end of the interview some patients asked me, "When is the interview going to start?" When I replied that it was already over, they were surprised.

Every time I got ready to see a new patient in my office or in the hospital, I remembered Sherlock Holmes' famous utterance in Sir Arthur Conan Doyle's 'The Adventure of the Abbey Grange': *"Come, Watson, come! The game is afoot!"* Though I did not have my own Dr. Watson to observe the unfolding drama, as a psychiatrist I was fortunate enough to lead as exciting a life as Sherlock Holmes did in London of Victorian times.

Patient's need versus my need: Early on in my practice a patient taught me that my priority must always be to meet the *patient's need* to have a trusting relationship with a compassionate doctor rather than *my own need* to make a quick diagnosis and offer definitive treatment. One morning shortly after starting my private practice, I went to the medical floor of the local hospital to see Dorothy, a 52-year old married woman, who had been admitted three days earlier for complaints of severe loss of appetite, as a result of which she had lost over 30 pounds in six months. The admitting physician found no physical cause for her malady and so he called me for a psychiatric consultation.

During the interview, Dorothy lay in bed looking outside the window and not communicating much. Instead of starting the interview by empathizing with her obvious feeling of hopelessness, I asked her a direct question, "What is bothering you?" Obviously, I was mostly interested in fulfilling *my need* rather than *her need* to find someone to entrust her life to. She must have sensed my selfish insensitivity. Looking away from me, she gave me one-word answers: Yes, no, sometimes. Frustrated by her what I considered as 'uncooperative behavior,' in her chart I declared her as depressed, prescribed her an antidepressant medication, and let her go home. I told her to make an appointment to see me in my office a week later.

Three days later the emergency room (ER) doctor of the same hospital called me to report that Dorothy was there having overdosed on the antidepressant medication I had prescribed. Those days the only group of antidepressant medications available was tricyclic. These drugs are very toxic, and often lead to death when patients overdosed on them. Obviously she had felt pretty hopeless after her disappointing contact with me. I told the ER doctor to admit the patient to the ward after appropriate treatment. I was very upset by the fact that the patient did not call me before attempting suicide. When patients do not call the doctor before attempting suicide, it is indicative of the fact that the doctor had failed to make *emotional connection* with the patient. Obviously, I had dropped the ball.

Somewhat disappointed with myself, I went to Dorothy's bedside and said empathically, "After our last meeting here, you must have felt totally hopeless." The patient nodded her head. I followed this with another empathic statement, "You must have felt that I did not care." Once again Dorothy nodded affirmatively. This mutual agreement connected us immediately. Now Dorothy was taking every volley I served.

"You must be going through a lot in life," I empathized. "I want to help you. I want to know more about your life situation. However, I cannot help you unless you tell me what is going on in your life. *I am a psychiatrist, not a mind reader. You've got to tell me!*"

This broke the ice. Dorothy let out a deep sigh, looked at me and smiled faintly. Then she opened up and began to pour out her heart out. She reported serious marital problems, conflicts with children and daughter-in-law, and many other stressful current and past events. Painful emotions accumulated in her mind till she felt, *"I just can't take it anymore!"* Once she opened up, she improved rapidly, and went home. I felt no fear that she would attempt suicide again, as I knew I had connected with her emotionally during the second hospitalization.

I saw Dorothy a week later in my office. She looked like a very different woman than the one I saw in the hospital. She was in good mood. She had gained some weight since her discharge.

Obviously, our emotional connection had made a big difference for her. She took out a neatly framed picture from a cloth bag. She had cross-stitched on a cloth, *"I am a psychiatrist, not a mind-reader. You've got to tell me!"* Signed D. L. Belcher 1983. Both of us had a good laugh. She said, "I am sure you have a lot of patients like me. They must know what I know now!" After a few more productive sessions, Dorothy moved on with her life.

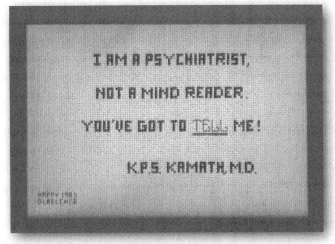

Picture#1: Dorothy's gift

I hung this framed picture prominently on the wall in my office waiting room till my retirement 27 years later, and it motivated thousands of people to open up to me in their very first contact.

Over the ensuing years since that incident, I continually raised my awareness about the power of empathy in developing *emotional connection* with my clients, and I placed the patient's need to have a trusting relationship with me over my need for a quick diagnosis and treatment. I realized that interviewing patients is like playing tennis. The patient serves the first ball by presenting his/her symptoms. If the psychiatrist fails to receive that volley properly, the patient would feel frustrated, and soon the game is over.

Here is one of many funny incidents I encountered in the course of my long practice, which shows how the *emotional connection* I made with a 'suicidal' patient gave me the confidence to send her home rather than hospitalize and drug her up:

A 60-year old woman walked into my office and asked my secretary if she could see me briefly. My secretary sent her to my office room.

"Hello, Dr. Kamath," she said. "Do you remember me?"

"I am sorry, I don't remember you."

"I am Pat. I saw you once 23 years ago!"

"Hi, Pat," I said smiling. "Nice to meet you again. Please take a seat. What can I do for you?"

"I just wanted to thank you for saving my life. When I saw you 23 years ago, I was about to end my life. I had held a loaded gun to my head many times. Then my friends told me to see you. That one session with you saved my life."

"Why did you want to kill yourself, Pat?" I asked curiously.

"Dr. Kamath, I found out that my husband was having an affair. When I confronted him, he blamed me for it. He said he wanted a divorce. I was devastated. I felt that I was responsible for the whole mess. I was inconsolable. I begged him not to leave me. He wouldn't budge. He filed for divorce. I felt so bad that I just wanted to die. When my friends came to know about my plan to kill myself, they forced me to see you."

"Then what happened?"

"Well, after listening to me patiently for 45 minutes, you wrote something on your prescription paper and told me, 'Go home and stick this prescription on your refrigerator. Read it every time you felt like killing yourself.' That piece of paper was on my refrigerator for ten years."

"Um!" I said. "What did I write on that piece of paper, Pat?"

"You wrote, 'Pat, you are not responsible for your husband's stupidity.'"

I laughed.

"You know, Dr. Kamath, before I came here, I was really scared to death that you would commit me to the psychiatric ward and drug me up. I have heard that that is what psychiatrists do to suicidal patients. I was truly surprised that you sent me home without a follow-up appointment. I felt so much better when I left your office, knowing that you would always be there for me if I ever needed you. I stuck your business card on the refrigerator with a magnet, and it is still on it!"

"Pat, thank you for telling me this interesting story. I am glad to see you doing well. "

"Actually, I am here because I brought my daughter to see you. She is going through some rough times. I know you can help her. Thank you, again. Bye!"

Guiding principles: My practice was based on four guiding principles: Unfailing *courteousness,* constant *availability,* professional *skill* and absolute *honesty.* I recommended these four principles to all unsuccessful businessmen I treated. I always told my patients what they needed to hear and not what they wanted to hear. I often heard my patients say to me, "My doctor told me to see you. He said you always tell it as it is to your patients." Thus I came to be known in the community by the epithet 'tells-it-as-it-is doctor.'

I treated every single patient as if he/she was my only patient, but I never got entangled with his or her personal issues. Patients often *transfer* on to the psychiatrist the anger they had toward important figures in their past, or they expect the psychiatrist to *fulfill their unmet needs* as children. While I connected with them emotionally by empathy, I scrupulously guarded my objectivity in making decisions. Because of this I was able to deal with even most difficult patients in their most difficult times. I established clear-cut boundaries between them and myself.

There were a few patients who did not let me connect with them. I realized that I could not help those who would not let me help them. A middle-aged man suffering from severe anxiety opposed every statement I made, every insight I gave him, and rejected every recommendation I made. After meeting with him three times, it became apparent to me that his only goal was to defeat me, and not to get well. I terminated him from my practice and returned the entire fee he had paid me. If a psychiatrist gets entangled with a patient such as this, he would lose the battle.

I have lost count of people who met me in shopping center or a public place or my office and said, "I am sure you don't remember me. I was your patient some years ago. You saved my life!" Yet, I had no memory of ever treating them, let alone saving their life.

What was important was that what little I said or did with kindness must have made a big difference in their life.

Here is one of numerous unsolicited letters I routinely received from my ex-patients in the course of my practice, which validates the above statement. What is important to note here is that this ex-patient did not have to write this letter, but he felt compelled to share his genuine feelings:

Dear Dr. Kamath,

I wanted to take this time to thank you for everything you have done for me in the past few months. I am sure you get many letters like this one, but to me this letter is special one. This letter isn't any more important because you have helped me more than you have helped many other people, but it is special to be because this letter is mine. I am sure you give all patients the same respect and consideration that you gave me, but you made me feel like I was the only patient you had while I was there. I remember the first day I came in to your office, life had never seemed more dim to me. However, after only a few minutes of listening to you, I felt an incredible relief because I knew there was at least one other person in the world that understood the way I was feeling. You have forever changed my life for the better, not just for this incident, but for future stress related problems as well. I will know the warning signs from now on, and anyone else I see having the same problems I was experiencing will also be able to benefit from the education I got from you. I will certainly recommend you to anyone I see suffering from the same problems

I was having. I would also like to thank you for considering cost while helping me. I am very aware of how I could have paid considerably more, but I don't feel I could have gotten any better help anywhere. Your help was such a small price to pay to have my life back the way I wanted it. Please accept my sincerest thanks for everything you have done for me. I will never forget what you have taught me.
Sincerely
Scott ____

What disabled people taught me: In addition to treating my private clients, in any given week I performed one-time psychiatric evaluation on 10 to 20 people for various agencies, such as Social Security Disability. They had all gone well beyond their breaking point, and they often suffered from multiple serious psychiatric and physical disorders. They considered themselves as totally disabled. Many of them had been through a grueling *medical wild goose chase* and had given up trying to get well, as they found no one who could help them. They felt totally hopeless in coping with their psychiatric disorders and life situation.

These demoralized patients taught me how their disorders progressed over the years from simple stress-related symptoms to serious intractable disorders, and how the baffled medical profession unwittingly contributed to their demoralization. Many of them suffered from *medical trauma* due to their painful experiences with medical professionals and hospitals, and *fear of medication* due to reckless prescription of drugs by inexperienced doctors and nurse practitioners.

Power of spoken words: Another thing my patients taught me was that every word I uttered, and its tone, mattered to them, and could have both positive and negative impact on them. A simple phrase, such as "I don't know" could be uttered in ten different tones conveying ten different messages. I often saw in my office patients devastated by a careless statement made by their exasperated doctor, such as, "I don't know what your problem is, lady. You need to have your head examined by a head shrink." The message is, "You are a hopeless case" or "You are a nut case." On one occasion I overheard an oncologist tell his terminally ill patient in the hospital, "Your cancer has spread everywhere. You have no more that two weeks to live!"

1. Here is one of many examples of positive outcome from a casual statement I made to a patient:

Susan, a 32-year old white woman, mother of a six-year old autistic child, came to see me for complaints of recurrent panic attacks characterized by sudden attacks of palpitation, shortness of breath, trembling of limbs, sweating, etc. lasting for a few minutes. Her panic disorder was caused by her on-going conflict with her domineering mother who constantly criticized her in regard to the care she gave to her six-year old autistic child. They clashed often. Susan experienced a lot of anger and guilt in her ongoing conflicts with her mother. However, she did not know how to deal with her mother without breaking up with her. She did not want that outcome. In other words, she felt trapped in her real life problem.

I put Susan on an anti-panic drug to control her panic attacks. Over the next year she improved a lot, and I saw her only once in six months. In her last visit with me, she reported doing very well, and she wanted to know how she could get off of her medications. She said, "I started feeling better after our last meeting six months ago. Something you told me helped me to solve my problem with my mother."

"Yeah?" I asked curiously. "What did I say?"

"You said, *'If someone repeatedly withdraws more from your emotional bank than deposits in it, close that account.'* I realized that every time I had any contact with my mother, I felt emotionally drained. So I told my mother on phone, 'Mom, every single time we talked, I felt emotionally drained. You make me feel like a bad mother. I am treating my child as recommended by his doctor. If you cannot say something positive about me in our conversation, I would rather you not say anything negative, or not call me at all.' Mom got all upset and said, 'In that case, I will not call you any more.' She has not called me in six months, and I have done perfectly well. I realized that she was too toxic for my wellbeing."

I told Susan how to taper off of her medication and call me if she had any problem in the future. I never saw her again.

2. Here is another case in which a simple statement made a big difference in resolving a father-son conflict: A businessman I met in a shop said that twenty years earlier he had brought his 16-year old son to me for a complaint of severe anxiety, characterized by shortness of breath. The boy's anxiety was related to an ongoing conflict he had with his soft-spoken father. Apparently the father did not approve of the "trashy girl" the son was dating at the time. The son rebelled and the father persisted in his demand

that he dump his girlfriend. The son did not want to upset his father, but at the same time he did not want to dump his girlfriend. His unexpressed feeling of being stifled by the father showed up as shortness of breath.

The businessman said that they both had a session with me regarding their conflict. He said, "Something you said changed everything in our relationship."

"Yeah? What did I say?"

"You said, *'Mr. G, you speak softly, but you come on like a steamroller.'* That woke me up. I realized that I was relentlessly breathing down my son's neck day after day though I never yelled at him. I realized that his anxiety and breathlessness had to do with my behavior. I backed off and my son did all right after that. Sometime later he dumped his girlfriend on his own. I want to thank you for helping me out."

3. Here is a case in which just two words I said in the interview made the patient very sick: A 35-year old woman came to see me for panic attacks. Toward the end of the interview while answering her question about the anti-panic medication I had prescribed, the patient became pale, began to tremble, felt nauseous, and said she was having a panic attack. She left my office abruptly saying she was too sick to stay any longer.

I saw this woman again three years later in my office. I asked her why she became sick when I saw her the last time. She said, "You said something that made me sick."

Surprised, I asked her, "What did I say?"

"While reassuring me about the drug you prescribed, you said *'Trust me!'* Those two words brought back bad memories of my uncle sexually abusing me when I was 10-year old. Before molesting me, he always told he, 'Trust me.' That is why I became very sick."

Obviously, this woman's panic disorder was actually part of her posttraumatic stress disorder.

Importance of education: Over the years, I realized that whereas the compassionate treatment they received helped my patients to recover from their emotional disorder, education about their psychodynamics helped them to stay well. At the end of the initial interview, I made patients sit in front of a big white board and wrote on it in detail how various bad events and problems caused them to experience various painful emotions, what mistakes they made in coping with them, how their symptoms appeared and progressed to the point when they came down with a stress disorder; and what they could do now to get well and stay well. I drew the picture of the balloon as representing the conscious mind, and soda bottle representing the hidden mind, and explained how they interacted. This audiovisual presentation in the very first interview helped them a great deal.

Seeing their life unfolding on the white board for the first time in their life, most patients felt so relieved that they broke down and sobbed. For the first time in a long time they knew exactly why they became sick and what they could do to get well and stay well. They felt as though they had just assembled the complicated jigsaw puzzle of their life. Their dreadful symptoms were no longer mysterious. After the initial reassuring and educative session, the relief they felt was glaringly obvious. People who practically crawled into my office, walked out feeling 'high.' Some of the 'high' feeling was due to the relief from fear of the interview with me. The following letter, which I received a week after the first interview, accurately reflects how most patients got immediate relief after the very first interview.

Dear Dr. Kamath,

I wish to express my sincere gratitude and great appreciation for your compassionate and excellent medical care and treatment. As you know from paying such careful attention to my history, you are very much aware of my long and most difficult suffering from Generalized Anxiety Disorder and Major Depression. I have been treated off and on for these illnesses for past twenty-five years. I have had hundreds of hours of therapy with at least two-dozen different doctors. None of them helped me very much. And not one, up until my visit with you last week, has even been able to describe or offer any effective treatment.

In less than one hour you were able to describe my exact symptoms and show a rational linkage to my painful early stress and later major depression and alcohol abuse. I have read and reread you wonderful book "Secrets of Stress Management," and find it to be of great comfort and help. I sent a copy to my wife Ellen in Maryland, and she also thinks it is of great benefit. I wish to buy two additional copies from you for a couple of close friends. Since my visit and talk with you I feel a little less stressed, and have in fact, as you promised, much better quality sleep...

Since my last visit I have not thought of suicide or craved alcohol, but I still have a lot of general anxiety...

Thank you and God Bless you for your good care.

Bill _____

Over 50% of new patients I saw were surprised to know that they did not have to come back to see me if they did the homework I assigned to them based on the education they received in the interview. The homework I gave them ranged from keeping a journal to writing an apology letter to visiting the grave of a loved one. The benefit of education often lasted forever. Many years after I last saw them I got unsolicited letters from my ex-patients expressing how they were able to live normal life by learning appropriate coping methods. Here is one of many letters I received just prior to my retirement from a patient I had no recollection of treating many years earlier. I have reproduced it here exactly as she wrote it:

Dear Dr. Kamath,

You may not remember me, considering it has been about 11 or 12 years since I last saw you, but I wanted to thank you for what you did for me. Before my mother brought me to you, because you helped out my older brother tremendously with his own panic attacks, I thought there was something terribly wrong with me. I would pass out, for what I thought was the most random reasons. Actually, I was just a young 18 year old girl who held everything inside until "balloon popped", as you used to say. I saw you for, I think, a little over a year. In that year, I learned how to deal with my stress and also eliminate my panic attacks. Since seeing you, I have not had another panic attack! Thank you so much for what you did for me and for helping to change my life.

You may be wondering, why now the email? Well, like I said, I was 18 at the time and I guess I didn't really appreciate how much you helped me. I am now, 31, and a friend of mine has a son that she thinks is having panic attacks. I instantly thought of you and referred her to you. I looked back over the years and saw how much you helped me and how you were God send. I had been to numerous doctors who said anything from brain tumor to putting me on seizure medicine. And of course none of those things were true or worked. Only you helped me and within a year I was a changed person. Not only that I had stopped passing out, but the way I dealt with situations and people around me.

Again, thank you. You will never know how much I appreciate the wonderful gift that you have of dealing with people who suffer from these issues!
God Bless,
Karen _____
Administrative Assistant

Public Education: To educate the public, I held regular public seminars on stress and stress-related disorders. From time to time I wrote articles in the local newspaper about these topics. The picture below appeared in Southeast Missourian daily newspaper on 8/14/1994 along with a big article. The paper's official photographer took it.

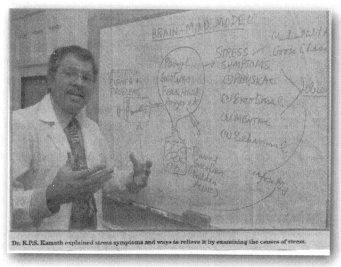

Dr. K.P.S. Kamath explained stress symptoms and ways to relieve it by examining the causes of stress.

Picture#2: Educating the public is equally important

Current State of the Art: To me personally psychiatry is more an art than a science. It used to be a *profession,* which healed people through empathy, analysis, insight and promotion of self-awareness. Today explaining patients' symptoms as caused by 'chemical imbalance' has become fashionable as well as immensely profitable to many recently trained psychiatrists as well as drug companies. Every year drug companies are coming up with newer drugs costing over 15 dollars a pill. Now psychiatry is almost exclusively a *business* of drug-treatment for quick relief of symptoms, and addition of more drugs for 'augmentation' when drugs are no longer effective. Thus 'drug-resistant disorders' have become fairly common. There are various contributing factors to this trend, such as promotion of expensive drugs by drug companies and the policy of health insurance companies to pay only for drug treatment. Now drug companies have taken over the task of 'educating psychiatrists' about the virtues of drug treatment. Handsomely compensated by drug companies, 'thought leaders' of psychiatry have been peddling drugs to their fellow psychiatrists claiming these drug treatments as 'the State of the Art.' This has suited many psychiatrists just fine, as discovering psychodynamics of patients is extremely complicated and time consuming for untrained doctors. They could make five times the money per hour by drug treatment as by psychodynamic analysis and therapy. This is the bitter truth few modern-day psychiatrists would admit to.

The flip side of this issue is, however, medicalizing psychiatry broke down the stigma of mental illness to a significant degree, and made more people to seek help for their psychiatric problems. However, this, too, has a flipside. Now physicians and nurse practitioners that have absolutely no clue about patients' psychodynamics are treating just about every symptom with psychotropic drugs. Very often they treat even normal grief with tranquilizers and antidepressant drugs, which suppress normal grief process. Most of these patients come down with serious psychiatric disorders sooner or later. Besides, widespread use of psychotropic drugs poses four serious public health problems:

1. Patients will have to deal with the serious side effects of drugs such as addiction, weight gain, diabetes, sexual problems, stroke, etc.

2. Rapid control of symptoms gives patients a false sense of security, which promotes *self-deception*. Instead of addressing their painful emotional issues, they go into a mode of *denial*, and think that their disorder was nothing

more than just a chemical imbalance. Painful emotions become buried in the hidden mind.

3. A later 'triggering event' could make these buried painful emotions to resurface suddenly and furiously, and precipitate a major psychiatric disorder such as suicidal depression or panic disorder, or even psychosis in vulnerable people. This might necessitate taking more drugs and for longer periods in the future.

4. Over time, more and more "drug-resistant" or "refractory" cases would develop.

The bottom line is that over the next few decades, more and more people would come down with more and more serious psychiatric disorders brought on by indiscriminate use of psychotropic drugs. The only good news is that people holding stocks in drug companies will retire comfortably.

Cookbook psychiatry: I will not be surprised if some recently trained psychiatrists would consider anecdotes I have presented in this book as pure fiction. If they do, that would be the undeniable proof of the depth to which psychiatry has descended as a profession. Perhaps they are content with practicing what I call cookbook psychiatry: Making a list of symptoms, arriving at a diagnosis based on the Diagnostic and Statistical Manual #5, ("According to this Manual, you have bipolar disorder"), and prescribing drugs recommended by drug companies for quick control of symptoms. Next patient please. The art of exploring their mind to figure out their deep-rooted traumatic emotional issues has fallen by the wayside. I say this after reviewing reports of numerous psychiatrists on the staff of reputable psychiatric hospitals, as well as those of privately practicing psychiatrists.

A good Office Manager: I cannot overemphasize the importance of the person who receives the phone calls of patients, and deals with referral agencies, in the success of a psychiatric practice. He/she is the face of every psychiatric practice. By the way this person interacts with the patients, one can tell the psychiatrist's true nature. I was truly blessed with a wonderful Office Manager who devotedly managed my office for 27 years till my retirement. She lived quite far from my office, and yet she managed to show up for work come rain, snow or ice storm, and she never missed a single day of work for any reason. With the exception of six-weeks long paid maternity leave, she never once took a sick-day leave. What I compensated for her invaluable service was never equal to what she contributed to my practice. She treated everyone with compassion and respect. My distraught patients often felt better after they talked with her just for a few minutes. She never got into an argument with a single patient. My patients loved her dearly. When I received letters of appreciation from my ex-patients or their relatives, they often included her name in them. Here is a letter from the daughter of an ex-patient who died of old age:

Dear Dr. Kamath,

I just wanted to express my sincere thanks to you and Kim for your care and concern for Betty down through the years. Betty loved you both and had such confidence in you. You were able to do what no one else could do- you turned her life around and helped her lead a productive one. You are not only an excellent doctor, but also a very special person, and Kim is like Family to everyone, always kind and caring.

I consider it a privilege to have known both of you.
Best Regards,
Kathy T.

Why did I write this book? When I opened my practice, knowing how anxiety-provoking it might be to prospective patients to see a psychiatrist, I printed a simple two-page *pamphlet* in which I presented my educational background, qualification as a specialist and my experience as a psychiatrist; fees I charged for my services, and policies I followed in my dealings with clients. I made sure that they encountered no surprises in their contact with me.

As years passed, however, I felt a need to add to this pamphlet more information about myself. I came to believe that my patients had the right to know me as a real person and not just a cardboard cutout in white coat. Since I could not do so in a small pamphlet, I created a separate *file* for the waiting room. It's main purpose was to inform my patients that like them, I, too, had gone through hard times in life; my life was an open book, and I welcomed them to get a glimpse into it.

Within a few years, this file swelled into a three-inch thick *folder* with the title, *"Just in case you are curious to know more about Dr. Kamath."* This folder included a three-page long autobiography. In it I described, with a map, the story of migration of my ancestors from Central Asia to India about 4,000 years ago as well as my own migration to America in 1970. I included in it photos of my great grandparents, my grandparents, my parents, my siblings, and my own family; newspaper articles about me, and written by me, and even photos of a Koi fishpond I had built with my own hands in my backyard. I left this folder on a side table in the waiting room of my office. I did not expect my patients to read it while waiting for their turn to see me, for I kept their waiting time not to exceed five to ten minutes.

To my pleasant surprise, my patients read the document with keen interest. When their turn came to see me, many of them said, "You go ahead and take others. I can't put this folder down!" Then another pleasant surprise: Those who read the folder seemed to be more open to revealing themselves to me when I interviewed them. It was clearly a *quid pro quo*. Many of them said something like, *"Dr. Kamath, I have never seen a folder like this in any doctor's office. Patients know so little about the doctors they entrust their life to. You should write a book about your life. It would make an interesting reading."*

An ex-patient's mother who read this office folder as well as my book titled 'Is Your Balloon About To Pop?' wrote from Florida:

> *"I think your clear and entertaining style of writing would really lend itself to another book with more anecdotes of your experiences with patients. Even if you have to kind of create composite individuals for the sake of patient confidentiality. And a nice picture of yourself would be good, too. As well as extended biographical information, like what you have in your office. Just a suggestion. I realize getting a book ready is monumental task, and I don't want to give you more stress… Sincerely, P.W.*

Thus encouraged by many patients, I decided to write this book after I retired from my practice in 2010. The sole purpose of this book is to educate people about psychiatry and human condition.

About this book: Over 39 years of my being in the field of psychiatry, I evaluated and treated thousands of patients, and it is impossible for me to write about all of them in a book such as this. Therefore, I have devoted the first few chapters of this book to only a few interesting case studies just to give the reader glimpses into the minds of patients who sought help for their intolerable suffering. These case studies also show how fulfilling the profession of psychiatry could be to those endowed with compassion, and devotion to helping distressed people. In addition, these anecdotes should give readers a glimpse into my everyday psychiatric practice. All names, of course, are not real names.

The chapters in Part Two of this book are devoted to almost insurmountable hurdles I had to overcome to achieve my American Dream as well as interesting encounters I had with various coworkers and hospitals.

About my earlier book: Readers curious to know more about how the mind works, and wanting to read additional interesting cases should read my book titled 'Is Your Balloon About To Pop?' subtitled, 'Owners' Manual for the Stressed Mind,' which I published in 2007 specifically for the benefit of my private clients. It describes in detail what stressed-out people could do to help themselves. This book is on amazon.com. Several thousand of my patients seemed to have benefited from that book. Several eminent psychiatrists praised this book as outstanding. Here is what a leading psychiatrist in the U.S. wrote immediately after reading this book:

> *Dr. Kamath,*   *February 25ᵗʰ 2009.*
> *I've started reading through your stress book and I have to congratulate you. It is really quite outstanding and a good read to boot. Is it available on Amazon or such so that I can recommend it to folks? You really have your finger on the pulse of clinical implications of current science.*
> *Chuck Raison MD*
> *Emory.*

About my name: My first name is Prabhakar, an ancient Indian name, which literally means, 'one who bestows light,' meaning, Sun. Early on, my American friends found it too tongue twisting. So they simply said, "We are going to call you 'Bob.' That Americanized name has stuck with me ever since. If I had a choice I would have said, "Call me Pubba." When people ask me, "How did Prabhakar become Bob?" I reply, "How did Richard become Dick? That is how."

With this rather lengthy introduction to my practice as well as my own mind, let me now narrate a few interesting case studies to illustrate the healing power of compassion.

CHAPTER 2

Small Acts of Kindness

THE OTHER DAY I INVITED my longtime friend and retired fellow physician, James Davidson, for dinner at my home. When I opened my private practice in 1982, his office was across the corridor from mine. Recalling the conversation we had when we first met in the corridor, he asked me, "Bob, do you remember what you said when I asked you, 'What do you do in your free time?'"

I confessed I had no recollection of our 34-year old conversation.

"You said 'I play God!'"

"Did I?" I said laughing.

To Jim, however, the phrase 'I play God' seemed to be no laughing matter. He must have taken it literally, and in its darker meaning, namely, doctors deciding whether a patient should live or die. Being a staunch Christian, he said that doctors have often played God in their dealings with seriously ill patients.

In the lively conversation that followed, I told Jim that I must have made a flippant remark when I said 'I play God,' for I had neither hubris nor delusion of possessing supernatural powers. I tried to explain what I meant by playing God.

"Jim, we all have the power to heal people with small acts of *kindness.* I believe that my small acts of kindness made a big difference in the life of my patients. That, in short, was what I must have meant when I said 'I play God.' We all have God within us, if only we let him manifest through small acts of kindness."

"That makes sense," said Jim. "However, it is easier said than done."

"Yes, indeed," I said. "To constantly remind me of the need for this quality in my interaction with others, I hung on the wall of my office room the utterance attributed to William Penn: *"I expect to pass through life but once. If therefore, there be any kindness I can show, or any good thing I can do to any fellow being, let me do it now, and not defer or neglect it, as I shall not pass this way again."*

"You know, Bob," said Jim, "Before you came to Cape Girardeau, we doctors had such a bad opinion about psychiatry. You brought dignity to your profession."

I thanked him for his kind words. Over the next three hours, between courses of spicy shrimp curry, chicken Tandoori, nan, lamb biryani and baingan bartha (egg pant dish), I briefly recounted several stories, which illustrated the power of kind acts in healing people. Now let me share with the reader some of those real life stories.

1. This incident happened some years ago. I was returning to America after visiting India. By the time my flight took off around 12.30 a.m. from Mumbai, I was exhausted. The chaos in Mumbai airport had taken its toll on me.

Shortly after the plane took off, the captain dimmed the cabin lights signaling that passengers could now go to sleep. It was amazing to see over 400 people, though packed like sardines in a flat tin can, already fast asleep. Even though my seat was too narrow for comfort, I closed my eyes, squirmed in it and tried to take a nap.

Two hours into the flight, an announcement on the intercom woke me up: "Medical emergency. Is there a doctor on board?"

As I was seated on the left aisle seat of the middle row, I quickly glanced from front to back to see if any doctor was getting up to assist the stewardess attending the sick person. I saw none. I was sure there were many "real doctors" on board since the flight was full, and its destination was Detroit, where a lot of Indian doctors practiced. Yet, no one came forward, perhaps because everyone was fast asleep. Or, perhaps, no one wanted to get involved.

I never missed an opportunity to help anyone in distress. So I got up and went looking for the spot where the emergency was. I didn't have to go too far. Just as I passed the cabin between my section and the one behind, I came upon the scene of the emergency. On the floor between the back wall of the cabin and the front part of the middle row of seats lay a frail, petite Indian woman in a large pool of blood. A tall, graceful but anxious blue-eyed blond stewardess stood over her holding a stethoscope tightly in both hands. She was anxiously scanning the plane's cabin to see if any doctor responded to the emergency.

As I came closer to the scene of the emergency, the stewardess scanned me to boot and asked, "Are you a medical doctor?"

"Yes, I am," I said. "What is going on?"

Looking at me somewhat skeptically, she asked, "May I look at your medical license, please?"

That was the last thing I expected from the stewardess in a medical emergency. However, I did not take this 'insult' personally, and rationalized that she was merely, 'covering her rear end,' as the saying goes. As we all know, in America frivolous lawsuits are commonplace. She was not going to take any chance with me.

I showed my credit card-sized medical license to her. She held the license in the dim overhead light and examined it closely. On it was written 'Physician and Surgeon' below my name. I did not tell her that I was a psychiatrist, and that I had forgotten how to attend medical emergencies except for helping someone choking on a piece of meat by applying the Heimlich method.

"This lady has been bleeding heavily," the stewardess said in a tone of exasperation. "Menstrual bleeding. Her husband says that she has been bleeding for three days and that she is on medication for it."

The Indian woman lying listlessly on the floor appeared scared to death. Probably she thought she was going to die any minute. Her forehead was dripping with sweat. The sari around her hip area, and the carpet beneath it were soaked with fresh blood.

I thought to myself, "What treatment can I offer a patient who is bleeding to death at 30,000 feet in the air, and 4000 miles away from the next stop -Amsterdam? The only thing I could do was to play God."

I knelt beside the frightened lady on the floor and introduced myself, "Hi there! I am doctor Kamath. What is your name?"

"Renu," she said in a feeble voice. In her faint smile I saw a flash of hope. Now a doctor was attending her!

"Renu," I told her in an authoritative voice. "Don't be scared. You will be all right, you understand?"

Renu smiled faintly, nodded her head and closed her eyes. She seemed to be rather dehydrated.

Renu's husband, an Indian in a dark three-piece suit, was sitting right there scared stiff.

"How long has she been bleeding like this?" I asked him.

"Three days," he said softly. "She was not bleeding when we boarded the plane."

"Is she on any medicine?" I asked.

"Yes."

"Do you have the prescription?"

He reached into the breast pocket of his coat and took out a prescription. I held it in the light and examined it. The entire prescription was written in Gujarati language, and I could not make head or tail of it. But wait! There was one word, just one word in English –Ergotamine. That was *the* medicine for Renu's problem –menorrhagia.

"When was the last time you gave her this medicine?" I asked the husband.

"Two hours ago," he said. "She is not due for another pill for four hours."

"Give me a pill," I said.

He reached into his coat pocket, took out a pill from a small bottle and gave it to me.

I asked the stewardess for a cup of water, which she fetched immediately. I put the pill in her mouth, lifted her head gently, and gave her a gulp of water to wash it down.

"Look here, Renu," I said while mopping her forehead with a towel. "You are on the *very best medicine* for this problem. I have given you an extra dose of it. It should start working in a matter of minutes. *There is absolutely nothing to worry about.* You will be all right in a few minutes. You understand?"

Renu gave out a deep sigh of relief and nodded again.

As I did this, a touching scene from my favorite movie Ben Hur (1959) suddenly flashed across my mind. In that scene, as Roman soldiers dragged enslaved Judah Ben Hur to the galleon, denied of water, thirsty and exhausted, he falls down on the ground saying, "God, help me!" Then a shadow appears over his body. It was the shadow of Jesus. With a water-filled gourd in his hand, Jesus kneels down, rubs Judah's face and forehead with some water, lifts his head, and gives him water from the gourd to drink. Judah regains his strength, gets up, looks at Jesus with gratitude, and is finally dragged away by Roman soldiers.

"Let her rest on the floor for a few minutes," I told the stewardess. "Give her plenty of fluids. Plenty of fluids! After a while you can put her back on her seat."

"OK. Thanks a lot, doc!" said the relieved stewardess, giving me a quick admiring glance. I went back to my seat and tried to nap once again.

One half hour later I went back to check how Renu was doing. Now she was fast asleep on her seat, leaning on her husband to her left. I felt her pulse. It was strong. Her husband appeared relieved. I reassured him that she would be all right, and that he should give her medicine as prescribed from now onwards with plenty of fluids.

Just as I turned to leave, the husband grabbed my hand and said, "Sir, in Amsterdam we need to get the connecting flight to Toronto. Our flight is not confirmed. Do you think we will get it?"

Obviously, in his helpless state of mind he thought that I could perform any miracle. Regardless, as if I had all the power in the world I played God once again. "There should be no problem whatsoever," I said. "As soon as you reach Amsterdam, ask for a wheelchair and an airport nurse to assist you. Take her to the ticket counter and tell them you must go to Toronto right away. They will do whatever to get you to Canada. Don't worry." He appeared immensely relieved by my reassurance.

I am certain that at least some of Renu's recovery was due to my small act of kindness. Giving people hope in the face of overwhelming distress does wonders. If I were not playing God here, what was I doing?

2. A doctor might not be able to play God all the time, but he could certainly play Angel. Here is how I played messenger of God with a terminally ill patient: Mary, a fifty five-year old married white woman, sat in front of me in my office looking extremely anxious. After acknowledging her anxiety with empathy, I asked her how I could help her. With tears in her eyes she said, "Doctor Kamath, honestly, I don't know what you can do for me. Two weeks ago my doctor told me that I have inoperable cancer of brain. It is very serious. He told me bluntly that I had about a month to live. I have been having severe panic attacks ever since. I don't want to die. This is such

a shock that I am not able to handle it. I can't sleep. I have no appetite. I have no energy. I am constantly anxious. I have panic attacks. I cry all the time. My doctor gave me alprazolam. It is not helping me."

Truly, what could I do to help a woman who knew she was going to die in two weeks? No drug could alleviate fear of impending death, unless that person is drugged-up to stupor. Only a power greater than myself could help her.

The surest remedy for extreme fear is Faith. Faith is a coping mechanism for the vast majority of people in this world. Belief that there is a higher power helps religious people to cope with even hopeless situations.

"Do you have Faith in God?" I asked her.

"Yes," she said. "I believe in Jesus. I have gone to church all my life."

"Where do people go when they die, according to your Faith?"

"They go to Jesus."

"Where is Jesus?"

"He is in heaven."

"How strong is your Faith in Jesus?"

"Right now, it is a little shaky."

"Do you know what Absolute Faith is?"

"No. I guess it is the Faith, which you do not question."

"Yes. You need to strengthen your shaky Faith and make it Absolute Faith."

"How do I do that, doctor?"

"Can I give you an example?"

"OK."

I told Mary the following story, which I cooked up on the spot: Two guys take a cab to go to the neighboring town. We will call the one with Absolute Faith AF, and one with Faltering Faith FF.

"What is your name?" AF asked the cab driver.

"God," said the driver. "Where do you want to go?"

AF told him where he wanted to go. As God drove the cab, both AF and FF noticed that God was driving recklessly through one red traffic light after another. While FF became scared witless, AF thought, "Well, God must know what he is doing." While AF fell fast asleep, FF became anxious and stayed awake wondering what would happen next. A short time later, suddenly the cab went off the road and began to go through a cornfield. AF woke up wondering what the commotion was, but thought, "God must know what he is doing," and went back to sleep. FF became even more anxious. He shouted to God, "What are you doing? Are you trying to kill me? Drop me off right now before I get killed!" God dropped off FF in the cornfield, and drove off with AF. Finally the cab reached the destination safely.

AF woke up, got off the cab, and asked God, "What do I owe you?"

"Nothing," said God. "You have already paid me with your Faith."

Mary listened to this story tearfully.

"Mary, you need to follow the example of AF. You need to constantly remind yourself that in two weeks, you *will be* with Jesus in heaven. You will be in His arms. When Jesus is carrying you, you should have no fear. Right?"

"I should not."

"Imagine how wonderful you might feel when Jesus, Son of God, is holding you in his arms and comforting you! You need to go home and pray to Jesus, 'Jesus, take me into your arms. I surrender my body and soul to you. I look forward to seeing you in two weeks!'"

"I can do that. I guess I should not have let my Faith lapse."

"Yes. However, it is never too late. You have been a good Christian all your life, right? This is the time you really need Jesus. I will give you some alprazolam to give relief from your anxiety. But nothing will help you better than Absolute Faith."

I gave her the copy of the poem, 'Footprints in the Sand.' The last verse in this poem went:

He (Jesus) whispered, "My precious child, I love you and will never leave you. Never, ever, during your trials and suffering. When you saw only one set of footprints, it was then that I carried you."

Mary gave out a deep sigh of relief and wiped her tears. She appeared significantly calmer. I told her to come back to see me in one week.

Mary did not show up for her appointment. A few days later I got a phone call from her husband.

"Doctor Kamath, Mary passed away yesterday," he said. "Ever since she saw you, she was at peace with herself. I want to thank you for helping her to deal with her terminal illness with her Faith rather than with drugs. She did not have to take her medicine as you prescribed it. I just wanted you to know. I wish there are more doctors like you who have Faith in Jesus."

I thanked the patient's husband for taking the trouble to call me, and said, "May Jesus give you the strength to bear with your wife's loss. Knowing that she is with Jesus should give you much solace."

During the course of my practice I often recommended my Christian patients teaching from the Bible. To women who wanted to punish their remorseful husbands for straying, I advised to take the high road: Mathew 5:39: *Show him the other cheek.* To those who suffered from feelings of sinfulness, I recommended Luke: 15:7: *I say unto you, that likewise joy shall be in heaven over one sinner that repenteth, more than over ninety and nine just persons, which need no repentance.*

Though I am not Christian by Faith, as a doctor it was my bounden duty to heal my patients with *whatever method that worked for them.* My belief or nonbelief in God or any religion should not be in the equation.

Everyone is entitled to hold on to one's Faith, which helps one to cope with life's miseries. The healer's job is to strengthen that coping mechanism, not weaken it.[8] Sometimes patients asked me, "Doctor, are you a Christian?" Invariably I answered, 'Well, I am a Christian in my heart. I practice Jesus' teachings. I guess that makes me a Christian, right?"

---

8 My own belief about gods and religion is similar to that of the Roman Emperor/ Philosopher Marcus Aurelius (121-180 C.E.): *Live a good life. If there are gods and they are just, they will not care how devout you have been but instead will welcome you based on the virtues you have lived by. If there are gods and they are unjust, you should not want to worship them. If there are no gods, you will be gone but will have lived a noble life that will live on in the memories of your loved ones.*

Just being there: Ever since I retired six years ago, numerous people have called me for advice. I had never met many of them. Just being there for people in distress does wonders. I recommend that readers watch the 1979 movie 'Being There.' In that movie a simple-minded, uneducated gardener by the name of Chance gives a dying tycoon solace *just by being there* for him during his last few days on earth. The movie ends with the scene in which Chance is shown walking on water. There was godliness in that simpleton. Now let me tell you how just being there for some people made a big difference in their life:

1. Four years after I retired, I received an email from a former patient of mine whom I had not seen in over 8 years. Here is the email exactly as she wrote it:

Hi Dr. Kamath-

I was your patient several years ago. I live in St Louis now and I'm having a very hard time. I was taking clomipramine for intrusive obsessive thoughts and anxiety, and was suffering from constipation so my new doctor, Dr. E. T. prescribed Luvox since I was having side effects. Luvox is terrible. The anxiety and obsessive thoughts have gotten worse and more violent and I'm unable to sleep. I met with him last week to explain what was happening and he kept me on Luvox and added Invega. The thoughts aren't going away and the anxiety is getting worse. I have a copy of your book and have been reading it most of the morning today. Do you still see patients? Is there anyone in St Louis you can refer me to? You were the only person who ever understood

me completely. I trust you and I know that if I could talk to you for a few minutes I would feel better. I tried to call your office and your voicemail said to email you at this address. I hope this note finds you and you will please give me a call. I will pay whatever you charge. Please call me if you are able at ___ ___ ___
Sincerely,
Kay.

The number Kay called was that of my home, and not my office, which I closed in 2010. I was vacationing far away from home when I received this email, and I could have ignored it on the pretext of having retired from practice four years earlier. Or, I could have emailed her, "I am sorry. I no longer have license to practice medicine. Go to the nearest emergency room." Instead, I called her immediately. Kay sounded extremely distraught. Even though I did not immediately recall who she was, I empathized with her suffering. It was obvious that her psychiatrist was young and inexperienced. I told her that clomipramine, a tricyclic drug, which she had been taking for over 8 years, should never have been stopped abruptly. Besides, taking Luvox while withdrawing from clomipramine would cause severe anxiety.

I told Kay to contact her psychiatrist and tell him what I told her. If he was not available, she could talk to her family physician and tell her what I said. I told her that since I had let my medical license lapse, I could not tell her what she should do with her medications, but I would gladly talk to her doctors on her behalf. I gave her my cellphone number and told her to call me any time day or night, or her doctors could call me anytime. I reassured her that she would be all right.

Kay wanted to know if I knew more experienced psychiatrist in St. Louis. I gave her names of two experienced psychiatrists in St. Louis, and offered to talk with either of them. Now that she had me standing by her, her insecurity and fear disappeared right away. Feeling much better, Kay thanked me and hung up. I sent her an email saying that I would gladly send her old medical records to her by priority mail if she sent me $10. I received the following email the very next day:

Hi Dr. Kamath :)

I can't tell you how comforting it was to hear your voice. You have helped me more than you will ever know. I truly believe you have saved my life more than once. I will send you $10 and the address to send my chart. I tried to get an appointment with the 2 doctors you recommended but they don't take my insurance. So, I went to the psychiatrist today who gave me the Luvox... and showed him your book (Is Your Balloon About To Pop?) and told him exactly what you told me to tell him. He has put me back on the clomipramine and I think I'm going to be ok.

Thank you again for your help and responding so quickly to my email. Here is a picture of me and my girls and my fiancé M. I thought you might enjoy seeing it.
I hope you are enjoying retirement and you are able to spend quality time and enjoy your family.
Take care,
Kay

I sent Kay her medical records by priority mail after returning home from vacation. She sent me a Thank You card with $10 check. She wrote:

> *Dr. Kamath, Thank you again for all of your help. You are a wonderful, caring, understanding and brilliant physician.*
> *I will never forget you.*
> *Sincerely,*
> *Kay.*

I had spent less than ten minutes on phone with Kay. Yet, it seemed to have made such a big difference in her life. I am quoting Kay's letters in this article not to toot my own horn but to emphasize how even a small act of kindness could make a big difference in the life of people.

2. Here is a small kind act, which made such a big impact on an ex-patient of mine: Five years after my retirement, I met my former patient Debra at Red Cross blood donation center. She said that she was doing well, but her sister Kendra, who was my client for almost 30-years, was going through some rough times. Apparently, Kendra was feeling a little depressed while withdrawing from a pain medication, which she had been taking for a few months postoperatively. She was already on a small dose of an antidepressant medication, which I had prescribed many years ago. Her orthopedic doctor suggested that she should switch to another antidepressant medication, which might help her pain better.

I had not seen Kendra for over 8 years. But I thought that switching her from one antidepressant drug to another was a bad idea, as most physicians do not know how to do it properly. As we read in the case of Kay above, most of them stop the old medication abruptly and start the new medication in big doses, leading to disastrous consequences. They do not know that drugs that work on the brain should never be stopped abruptly. So I told Debra that perhaps just increasing the dosage of the medication she is already on might be a better idea. "Tell Kendra to talk to her family doctor about this," I said. "He can call me if he has any question." That was all I said.

Two months later I got the following letter from Kendra:

Dear Dr. Kamath,

This note is two months late —that means I am doing well! I can't thank you enough for almost 30 years of your expertise and support. Debra (my sister) and I have had much more contended, productive lives thanks to our association with you.

Your advice to simply increase my current Rx to see me through the withdrawal of Percocet was also absolutely 'spot on!' I did talk with/see Dr. J.M. as you advised and he and I sang your praises.

Thank you again for being the wise and trusted physician who has changed my life immeasurably.
Fondly,
Kendra.

3. Recently an ex-patient of mine I had not seen for over ten years, -I have no idea who she is- called me complaining

of severe anxiety. I listened to her patiently for five minutes and told her to read the first chapter of my book. I told her to search for the cause of her anxiety, and that she needed to adjust her medication a little bit. I told her to contact her doctor, and tell him to call me if he had any question about it.

Two weeks later I received an expensive 'Thank You' card from that woman. The front cover of the card said, "You Care… and It Shows." Inside it said, "You're the kind of doctor who treats the person as well as the patient." This was followed by the patient's handwritten note, "I'm feeling better thanks to your advice. I greatly appreciate your taking the time to help me. L. W."

Honestly, I have no idea what I did to deserve this Thank You card. Obviously, whatever little I did meant a lot to this woman in distress.

4. In 1973, when I was getting "non-existent training" as a second year Resident in psychiatry, I was assigned to see some patients in an Outpatient Clinic. As I knew nothing whatsoever about psychiatry, psychodynamics or psychotherapy, I just kept my mouth shut and listened to the patients who came to see me week after week.[9] My patients did not know that they were talking to a total idiot. However, they came week after week, and poured their hearts out to me. I was afraid to say anything lest

---

9 Some time later a senior Resident psychiatrist told me that people rarely keep their appointments regularly.

I might say something stupid. 44 years after my stint at this clinic, I still remember a patient by the name of Sarah who came just to shed tears of sorrow over something. Gradually, they all felt better. It dawned on me that very often nodding your head understandingly and saying nothing is better than saying something stupid that could make matters worse. When I asked them what made them feel better, they all said they felt better just knowing I was there for them. The lesson I learned from this was that it takes so little outside help for some people to heal themselves. They just need a listening post. I always recommended my patients to go for long walks with someone who would listen to them without interrupting, judging, criticizing or advising.

CHAPTER 3

Mending Broken Hearts

PSYCHIATRY IS MOSTLY ABOUT MENDING broken hearts. As a practicing psychiatrist, my business was to help people in a great deal
of pain, both emotional and physical. Often the patient's main
physical symptom was the symbol of his/her emotional pain.
In other words, the body weeps if the mind refuses to weep. If
patients seek help immediately after the symptoms appear, they
could be "cured" of their malady promptly. If not, these symptoms could become chronic, and cure becomes more difficult to
achieve, as we will read in the next chapter. Here are two case
studies of patients who benefited immediately from release of
their inner painful emotions:

1. I was fast asleep at home when the telephone rang around
   5.30 a.m. It was the head nurse of Emergency Room
   (E.R.) at the local hospital.

"Good morning, Dr. Kamath. This is Southeast Hospital E.R.
nurse. Dr. Thomas would like to talk to you."

Dr. Thomas said that he wanted to admit Monica, an 18-year old white single woman, to the psychiatric ward. He gave me the following story: Monica's friends had brought her to the E.R. saying she had gone blind after she hit her head to the bar over her bunk bed in her dorm. He did a C/T scan, which came back as normal. He called in the ophthalmologist on call for an opinion on this case. This specialist examined Monica and declared that he found nothing wrong with her eyesight. But Monica said she could see absolutely nothing.

"This is a case of conversion reaction," said Dr. Thomas. "I think she should be on your floor."

"Conversion reaction" is a condition in which painful emotions are expressed in the form of a bodily symptom.

"Go ahead," I said. "I will be there shortly."

"The game is afoot!" I said to myself.

Before leaving home I grabbed my video camera to record the drama that I knew would unfold during the interview. When I entered Monica's room, she was in the hospital gown, sitting propped up against the back of the bed. She was a slightly plump white woman with an expressionless face, looking straight at the front wall, so characteristic of really blind people. She did not acknowledge me when I entered her room. When I introduced myself she did not turn her head to look at me but merely offered me her right hand. I asked Monica if she would mind if I recorded the interview on a camcorder. She said she did not mind.

I spent the first ten minutes primarily getting to know Monica and how her blindness developed. She said she was a freshman at the local university, living in the dorm. Early that morning when she got up from her bunk bed she banged her head against the bar over the bed. Shortly after that one of her eyes became blurred. Within 30 minutes her other eye also became blurred. Within an hour she went completely blind in both her eyes. Alarmed by the seriousness of this symptom, her friends decided to take her to the E.R., but she demurred. She said, "I didn't think it was a big deal." In any case, her friends "forced" her to go to the E.R., and here she was a reluctant patient. She had a similar episode of blindness a couple of weeks earlier, but it had cleared up without medical treatment.

Monica had left home for college in August of the previous year. Between then and February of this year, she had been under a lot of minor stresses such as sprained ankle, a bout of cold, etc. She had been coping with her stress by drinking alcohol. I empathized with her and avoided asking any direct questions. Once I felt that I had the good *emotional connection* with Monica, I decided to probe her mind a little more vigorously.[10] Feeling assured that I had all the time in the world to listen to her story, Monica gave me the following story:

Monica's parents lived in a small town over 250 miles from this town. Her father, a retired police officer and Baptist minister, was seriously ill with diabetes and heart disease. He was going blind on account of his diabetes. Over the past few weeks, Monica's mother had been calling her to report that her father's health was getting worse and his doctors had not been helping much. Sometimes he coughed incessantly and choked on the

---

10 This emotional connection with the patient is often referred to as 'therapeutic alliance.' This term means that the doctor and the patient are working together to solve the patient's problem.

mucous in his lungs. Monica constantly worried that he might die any time. She felt that her mother was not doing enough to get her father the needed medical care, but felt *totally helpless to do anything.*

Monica's relationship with her father was very bad till just a year earlier. She hated him and everything he said and did. She did not know why she hated him, but when she turned 17, she decided to make up with him, and make him be proud of her. By the time she left for college in August, she felt very close to him.

Two months back Monica went home for Christmas holidays. When she knocked on the door, her father opened it, moved his head to six inches from her face and asked, "Who is it?" Monica was so heartbroken over his poor health that she spent the entire Christmas holidays worrying over her father's declining health.

When Monica returned to college in January, she was not the same. She felt anxious and depressed. She slept fitfully through the night. She suffered frequent bouts of headache. She coped with her emotional pain by drinking beer. She could not share her emotions with anyone as her father had raised her to "be strong." She thought that expressing her grief to anyone was a sign of weakness. Now she felt so *helpless to do anything* about her father's health problems, and she often felt "I just couldn't take it anymore!"

As Monica began to open up to me, her face became flushed and eyes became tearful. Telling me all this, she sobbed uncontrollably again and again. I held her hand to comfort her and wiped her tears with tissue paper. I acknowledged her sadness over her father's plight and her *helplessness to do anything* about it. As she told me her heartbreaking story, emotions began to return to her formerly bland face. She kept repeating, "I felt so helpless because I just couldn't do anything for him!"

When she calmed down a little, I said to her gently, "Monica, *you are doing something for him, you know?*"

"What am I doing for him?"

"You are suffering for him. You are suffering the same blindness he is suffering from."

"What are you telling me?"

"I am telling you that because you cannot do anything for him, you are giving him company by going blind yourself. What more could you do than to go blind for your father whom you love so much?"

"The thought occurred to me that I might be going blind because of his suffering. I don't want to go blind," Monica said sobbing and trembling. "I want to be able to see well again."

"You won't go blind, Monica," I assured her. "You will get completely well. But you must learn to talk about whatever is bothering you and express your emotions like you did just now."

Monica nodded her head.

"Monica," I said. "Can you look at me?"

Monica turned her head to look at me.

"Can you see me? What do I look like?"

"I can see you. You are dark. You have a mustache."

"Good. Your eyesight is coming back."

"What do I do now?" Monica asked.

"Cry a little bit more! Because you are hurting like hell, and because you won't let your emotions flow out, your body is doing it for you. So from now on you will have to start talking about your feelings freely. Give up being strong and learn to fall apart. Is that a deal?"

She took my extended hand and nodded affirmatively.

"I can see very clearly now." Monica turned her face to look out of the window at the beautiful, crisp February morning.

"Isn't the world out there beautiful?" I said.

"Yes, it is!" Monica was smiling with happiness at the return of her eyesight.

"Isn't that a miracle? Sort of?" I said in jest.

"Yes, it is!" said Monica giggling. "You do this all the time?"

"I do this all the time," I joked.

"What is your name?" asked Monica.

I told her my name and said I would be back to see her the next day. I went on to make my rounds of the ward. Well, in ten minutes, the nurse came to me to report that Monica was all dressed-up to go back to her dorm. I said I had no problem with it. The nurse gave Monica an appointment to see me in my office the following week.

When I saw Monica in my office four days later, I could not recognize her. She was a beautiful woman, very pleasant and full of smiles. She said that after she left the hospital her mother called to say that a whole new team of doctors had taken over her father's treatment and that he was doing better. She said that the whole experience of going blind and regaining her eyesight gave her the *insight* into her own mind. From now on she would become a more "self-aware" person and make every effort to share her emotions with a confidant. She would avoid using denial and drinking alcohol as her coping mechanisms.

I never saw Monica again. She kept in touch with me occasionally by writing letters. Three and one half years later, I received the following letter from Monica:

Dr. Kamath,

Just wanted to let you know how well I am doing. Currently I am in the process of testing for the Missouri State Highway Patrol. I signed the releases because I didn't think they would have any bearing on my being selected for the academy. I am very excited about this part of my life.

In August I went to alcohol rehabilitation classes/counseling. Dealing with the fact that I had a drinking problem really helped me. I have been sober and drug-free since I left Cape Girardeau in May.

Currently I am a youth chaperone, and Choir Director at New Life Church. I am a Certified Nurses Aide at a Nursing Home and of course a testing applicant for the State Patrol.

I feel like a new person —I am a new person. I hope you can share the news of success to your classes. Thank you for talking with me and for giving me a chance to help others.
Sincerely,
Monica

Monica gave me permission to show her video to people who attended my stress management classes.

What happened here? If we were to compare Monica's mind to a balloon, by the time she was hospitalized, it was filled with so many painful emotions that it was about to pop. That is why she kept saying: "I just can't take it anymore!" However, her belief that expressing her emotions was a sign of weakness made her clam up. She coped with her extreme feelings of helplessness by going blind herself as a sign of solidarity with her ailing dad. By using empathy as a tool, I broke down Monica's denial, raised her awareness of her pent-up grief, and facilitated its expression. Her balloon shrank and her symptoms disappeared, and she developed insight into her malady. She probably had many old emotional issues in her hidden mind, but this was not the time to bring them up. I educated her about the importance of expressing her painful emotions.

This is a classic example of how in many cases prompt intervention could get patients well immediately and prevent *medical wild goose chase.* In this case, the patient was open to insight and benefited from it. If Monica was close-minded, this intervention would have failed, and she would have gone on a medical wild goose chase, and ended up with *disillusionment, disgust* and *demoralization.*

The question is, what would have happened to her blindness had she not gotten treatment right away? Many Cambodian women developed similar blindness after witnessing Khmer Rouge atrocities on their children. As they did not get timely treatment, their retina degenerated, and they suffered from permanent blindness.

When a body organ is not used, it atrophies due to disuse. There are instances of atrophy of limbs of people suffering from paralysis of an arm or leg as a result of not getting prompt treatment for their 'conversion disorder.' This term means, unexpressed painful emotions become converted into a physical symptom. Once the physical symptom becomes chronic, it is extremely difficult to treat it. Fear of losing disability payments, and losing sympathy of others if one got well, lead to persistence of the symptom. This is called 'secondary gain' phenomenon.

2. Now let us review how one could experience severe emotional pain as severe physical pain, and how insight into this phenomenon could cure that pain immediately.

One afternoon when I was busy seeing patients in my office, I got a frantic phone call from the chief nurse on the third floor of the local hospital, of which I was a staff member. She wanted me on the floor right away to see a 43-year old woman who was screaming with pain in the chest. No amount of morphine given could alleviate her pain.

"Please hurry up," said the nurse. "We just don't know what to do any more!"

I could hear the patient's screams in the background before the nurse hung up the phone. Telling my patients in the waiting room that I had an emergency in the hospital, I left.

When the elevator door opened on the third floor of the hospital, I could hear blood-curdling screams in the corridor. The nurse was waiting for me outside the patient's room. When I entered the patient's room, there were six people around the patient, including the patient's husband, helplessly watching her.

The patient on the bed was a brunette white woman in the hospital gown. Her eyes were closed and she was screaming as if someone was sticking a knife into her chest. Sometimes she arched her body up from the bed like a bow, screaming loudly, "My God! I just can't take this pain! Do something, damn it! Help me!"

I went straight to the right side of the patient's bed, took Sandy's right hand in mine and introduced myself. I asked all of the attendants to leave the room except for the nurse and the patient's husband. I started the conversation by empathizing with her chest pain, "Sandy, you are hurting like hell, aren't you?"

"Yes!" Sandy said. "Do something, quick!"

"How long ago did you give her a morphine shot?" I asked the nurse.

"Just ten minutes ago."

"Good," I said. "Sandy, it should start working any time now. How long have you suffered pain like this?"

"Three days!"

"Oh, my God! You have been suffering like this for three days?" I empathized.

Sandy's husband intervened and said, "Since her father died three days ago, right on this ward."

"Oh! I am sorry to hear that, Sandy. That must have hurt you like hell."

Sandy nodded, with her eyes still closed. Her eyes were now moist. I squeezed her hand tight and said, "Sandy, you must have been very close to him. You miss him very much, right?"

Sandy nodded again, and started sobbing.

"Sandy, what did your dad die from?"

"Cancer. He had lung cancer. They operated on him a couple months ago. Then he developed pleural effusion. They had to drain fluid from his lungs by sticking a big tube into his chest."

Sandy moved her left hand to the right side of her chest and pressed it as if she was hurting real bad.

"So he must have suffered a lot of pain before he died," I said.

By now Sandy was sobbing uncontrollably.

"They stuck this thick tube into his chest! Oh, my God! Oh, my God. It must have hurt him like hell!" Saying this Sandy pressed her left hand over the right side of her chest as though she was suffering the same pain as her dad did when doctor placed the plastic tube into his chest.

"Sandy, you are hurting at the same place where they stuck the tube in to your dad's chest."

"Yes, yes! I just couldn't see him suffer pain like that day after day. Every time I entered his room, he cried in pain. No one did anything to help him. He cried, and I cried helplessly with him. I just could not take it anymore!"

"You felt totally helpless to do anything for him, didn't you?"

"Yes. I felt so helpless. There was nothing I could do. Day-after-day he suffered pain, and more pain. I just could not take it anymore!"

Now Sandy was pouring her heart out freely. Tears were pouring profusely out of her eyes and nose. I held several paper towels to her nose and told her to blow her nose. Sandy kept crying like this for the next fifteen minutes. After each sobbing episode she took a deep breath.

"When he finally died, I thanked God. I felt bad for wishing death on him, but I had no choice. I wanted his suffering to end."

"You felt terribly guilty for wishing him death, right?"

"Yes."

"Sandy, your guilt prevented you from grieving over him. I bet you did not cry when your dad died, right?"

"Yes. I just could not cry."

"Sandy, I don't blame you for wishing him death. He was terminally ill, and the sooner his misery ended, the better for him, right? When people don't grieve over death of a loved one, sometimes they suffer from the same symptom as the dead person. Now that you are more aware why you have this pain, and you have talked and cried about your dad, how is your pain?"

"It is better! Almost gone!" Now Sandy managed to smile a little.

"Isn't this a miracle?" I said in jest.

"Yes, it is!" said Sandy.

"Sandy, if you continue to grieve like this, and express your emotional pain, your chest pain will go away completely."

Sandy opened her eyes and smiled incredulously. "Really?"

"Yes. But I want you to remember your dad and continue to grieve. When you return home today, you should look at your dad's photos and remember all the good and bad stuff about him, cry and sob and let it all go. Make an appointment to see me in my office in a week. We will take it from there."

"Yes, I feel better already. Can I go home right now?"

The patient's incredulous husband and the nurse were anxious to end this drama as soon as possible. Immediately thereafter, the nurse pulled out the patient's I.V., told Sandy to dress up, and had her sign the discharge papers.

I saw a totally different-looking Sandy in my office a week later. She said she was back to being herself. I told her jokingly, "Now get out of here! I don't want ever to see you in the hospital or in my office again. You hear me?"

Sandy had a good laugh. Thanking me profusely, She left my office.

What would have happened if Sandy did not get timely help? If untreated promptly, many patients such as Sandy end up becoming chronically ill with pain somewhere in the body, or they cope with their emotional pain by burying it deep into their *hidden mind*. When they do that, pain goes away, and over time they forget the painful event and move on with life. However, such buried emotional pain of an old wound could resurface suddenly triggered by a similar current painful event. I call this phenomenon *double whammy*.

In the next chapter let us study cases of two women who buried their emotional pain in their hidden mind, and moved on with their life. However, their repressed emotional pain resurfaced later on as physical pain triggered by another event, leading to a fruitless medical wild goose chase.

CHAPTER 4

Medical Wild Goose Chase

AT ANY GIVEN TIME, THERE are thousands of people in America making rounds with doctors and hospitals looking for cure for their chronic physical symptoms such as pain somewhere in the body, dizziness, heart flip-flopping, bouts of diarrhea, etc. If someone tells them that their physical symptom is due to their unexpressed emotional pain, they deny it, or even get very angry. Not knowing that the brain/mind/body is one indivisible unit, they think they are being accused of faking or imagining their symptom. Doctors have little awareness of the phenomenon of *medical wild goose chase,* and they unwittingly contribute to the pathology by drugging up patients. A lot of Pain Clinics have sprung up across America to treat patients suffering from chronic pain somewhere in the body, and are raking money like we rake leaves in autumn. In many of these patients, *secondary gain* is the reason for the persistence of their symptoms. Medical wild goose chase has contributed a great deal to the skyrocketing cost of healthcare in America.

Resurfacing of painful emotions related to past traumatic experiences is the cause of persistent physical symptom of patients going on medical wild goose chase. These patients had always dealt with their emotional pain by being stoic, and they buried them in their hidden mind. When they were going through traumatic experiences, they simply said to themselves, "I will not think about it or talk about it. I will just forget about it."

Let us examine two cases of chronic pain resulting from the 'blast from the past,' which could have been avoided by timely intervention.

1. Janet was a 56-year old white widow, mother of two grown children. She was an elementary school teacher before she went on Social Security Disability about a year ago. She looked rather apprehensive as she entered my office. Her greying hair and facial lines gave me the impression that she had suffered a lot in life. She looked much older than her 56 years. She shook my hand gently, did not smile, and sat on the edge of the chair I offered her as if she wanted to get out of my office as soon as possible. She glanced around my office as if to check if there were any video cameras recording the interview. Not seeing any, she became a little relaxed.

Janet's internist had briefed me about her ordeal before she showed up at my office. She had suffered from severe pain over the upper right side of her abdomen –over the gall bladder area- for two years. She had seen many doctors and had undergone many surgeries for the relief of her pain. He was concerned that she was abusing narcotics he prescribed her. Over the past year the number of narcotic pills she was taking daily had increased significantly, and he felt he could no longer enable her narcotic abuse.

Before beginning our conversation I noticed that Janet gently pressed with her left hand the area over the right upper quadrant of her abdomen –the area over the liver- as if to relieve her pain.

I started our conversation by empathizing with her pain and suffering: "Looks like you are hurting a lot over your liver area, aren't you?"

Such genuinely empathic statement addressing patient's suffering usually has dramatic effect. Janet became tearful instantly, and gave out a big sigh. It was a sigh of relief that said, *'This man understands my pain.'* Probably she expected me to hassle her with the issue of narcotic abuse.

"I am told you have been through a lot with doctors and hospitals over the past two years."

I was referring to the medical trauma she had experienced while on her medical wild goose chase. Once again, Janet gave out a deep sigh and became tearful in response to my empathic statement. I moved the tissue paper box towards her and said, "Here, take this." Janet was obviously embarrassed by her breakdown. She plucked two tissue papers abruptly from the box and pressed them against her tearful eyes.

"I was determined not to do this," she said. "I am not the one to complain, you know. I am not a whiner."

"You have always tried to cope with life by being strong, haven't you?" I acknowledged.

"Yes, always," she said. "That is why I don't understand why I have to see you. I am not imagining this pain. I am not faking it. I am not crazy. I know you run a stress clinic. Other than the stress of living with this severe pain, everything is all right in my life. I can't complain."

"No one can imagine or fake pain such as yours," I said with much compassion. "No one would take narcotics for pain that does not exist."

Janet nodded her head in agreement.

"Tell me, how did your pain start and what ordeals have been through in the past two years."

"Well, it is a long story. I don't know if you have the time to listen to all this."

"I have all the time in the world for you. I really want to know about your suffering."

Janet told me the following story: About two years ago, overnight she developed severe pain over the right upper abdominal (liver) area. Her *Medical Wild Goose Chase* began right away.

1. First she ran to the local emergency room. After several tests, the E.R. doctor told her he found nothing to explain her pain. He told her to see her Internist.
2. Suspecting that she might have some type of gall bladder inflammation her Internist ordered many more tests. Urine and blood tests, and MRI scan were normal. Her doctor sent her to a general surgeon.

3. Janet's pain in the liver area baffled the surgeon. He felt it was necessary to perform "exploratory surgery" on her to rule out malignancy of some kind. He cut her open and found nothing in the liver or gall bladder to explain her pain. He removed her gall bladder, just in case. Following surgery, Janet's pain continued. The surgeon sent her to a neurologist.

4. The neurologist ordered a few more tests, most of them had nothing to do with her pain, and after he had milked her insurance, he referred her to a neurosurgeon for a 'second opinion.'

5. The neurosurgeon could not find anything to explain her pain. He told her that he could cut off the nerve supply to the liver area, which should help. So the patient underwent rhizotomy (cutting off of nerves at the point they come out of the spinal cord). This did not alleviate her pain. The exasperated neurosurgeon threw up his hands and sent her to a famous medical center 'for further evaluation.'

6. At the major medical center, another neurosurgeon came up with a brilliant idea. Why don't we just cut off pain conducting nerve fibers in the spinal cord itself? The patient said that she was a game for it. By now Janet was so frustrated that she was willing to do anything to alleviate her chronic pain. So this neurosurgeon cut the nerve bundles in the spinal cord, and said, "Well, you are cured!" The patient's pain continued. The doctor was floored. He sent the patient to another famous medical center.

7. A 'team of doctors' at this center reviewed all the tests once again. Not finding any cause for the patient's pain, it did the next best thing –psychiatric consultation.

8. A young psychiatrist wearing a French-cut beard interviewed her for fifteen minutes, made a list of symptoms, and diagnosed her as suffering from 'chronic pain syndrome' and 'major depression.' Both these are garden-variety diagnoses, which stand for 'I don't know what the hell is going on with this lady!' When psychiatrists feel this way, which is almost 99% of the time with patients such as this, they drug them up. Few modern psychiatrists have either the time or the interview skill or patience to make patients such as Janet open-up. Their primary goal is to meet their own need, namely, make a diagnosis based on a list of symptoms and offer drug treatment.

9. Janet came back home hurting more than ever before, and feeling very depressed. By now, one half million dollars had been spent, almost none from her own pocket, and there was nothing to show for it.

10. By this time Janet suffered from what I call Three Major Ds: Disillusionment, disgust and demoralization –a deep sense of hopelessness.

11. Unable to return to work as a schoolteacher, Janet reluctantly applied for Social Security Disability (SSD). She got approved promptly when the disability evaluator saw three feet high stack of medical records from reputable doctors and hospitals. Normally approval for

disability payments would take three years and several 'second opinions,' not to mention a court appearance with a 'team of lawyers.'

12. Janet had agreed to see me only out of fear that her Internist would cut off her supply of pain pills if she refused. She was afraid that either I would declare her as insane or a faker. If I declared her as a faker, she risked losing her SSD checks. By now 'secondary gain' had set in, and treatment would be very difficult.

During the entire narration of this horror story I acknowledged her frustration as well as suffering by means of nodding and occasional words of empathy such as, "You must have been thoroughly disappointed and disgusted by all this runaround," and "By now you must have felt quite hopeless and helpless." All the while, I was raising the patient's awareness of her inner pain. The patient must have noticed genuine empathy I felt for her physical pain as well as her fruitless and painful rounds with doctors, hospitals, laboratories and pharmacies.

Now that I had made the emotional connection with Janet, I ventured to explore deeper into her mind. However, it would have been futile for me to ask direct question such as, "Tell me what kind of stress you were under before your pain started?" Such direct questioning invariably obtains a reply, "Everything was great in my life!" So I applied 'stealth interview' technique.

"Janet, where were you born and raised?"

"In Gordonville. Not far from here."

"What did your parents do for a living?"

"They were both farmers. They have both passed away."

"Did they raise you?"

"Yes. I had good childhood."

"Where did you go to school?"

"I went to the Jackson High School. Then I went to the local University. After graduation, I became a teacher. That is all I have done till I went on disability. Elementary schoolteacher. I liked my job very much."

"How old were you when you got married?"

"I was eighteen, right out of high school. That was what all girls did then. My husband was a plumber."

"How many children do you have?"

"I have two boys. One is thirty three and the other is thirty."

"How are they doing? Are they in good health?"

"My older boy is doing well. My younger son's health is not good."

"Really? What happened?"

"Two years ago, he was in a motorcycle accident. The motorcycle skidded on an icy patch, and his trousers got caught in its wheels. It dragged him two hundred feet with him. He broke his leg and ankle, and he was in the hospital for over two weeks. He has not been able to work regularly since."

"Oh! What a tragedy for a young man to suffer!"

"Yes," Janet agreed. "The state patrol woke me up at 2 in the morning and dropped this bomb on me. I dressed up as fast as I could and rushed to the hospital."

"Must have been a scary deal!"

"Yes. At first I thought he died or something. As I came on the floor where my son was, I heard him wailing and screaming, 'Help me! Help me! I am hurting. Give me a shot! Nurse, please! I can't stand it!' I rushed to his bedside and was shocked to see his leg in the cast, dangling from the rod above. He had already undergone surgery. He was all banged-up from the accident. His eyes were swollen and his face was cut up in many places. I could hardly recognize him. He kept pleading with me to tell the nurse for morphine shot. I felt so helpless, so helpless!"

Janet was sobbing softly as she told me this horror story. She picked up more tissue paper to blow her nose.

"I was totally stunned by the whole scene. After consoling him for a while I went home and went to bed." I slept fitfully for a couple of hours. Then I woke up around 5 a.m. with severe pain on the right side of my stomach. I thought I was going to die. So I ran to the emergency room. I have never been the same since."

"Is your son doing better now?"

"Well, John has been out of work since the accident. I have had to support him. He has recovered some since then. He is trying to go back to work."

"When did you lose your husband, Janet?"

"Well, he died twenty two years ago. My boys were 11 and 8 years old."

"Oh, what a loss it must have been for a young family!"

"Yes. He suffered a lot before he died."

"What happened?"

"He was diagnosed with terminal liver cancer. He did not live long after he was diagnosed. Doctors said there was nothing they could do for him. So they sent him home. He suffered a lot of pain though."

"How did he cope with it?"

"How could one cope with severe pain?" Janet said pressing her left hand over her liver area. "Those days doctors were very strict with pain pills. He screamed and yelled begging me for pain pills and injections. He screamed, 'Help me, please, Janet! Please give me a shot! Help me!' I felt so helpless. I didn't know what to do. I put him in a room and just shut the door. My kids were very upset hearing his screams. So I stuffed their ears with cotton swabs to muffle his screams. Those were horrible days for me."

Janet shuddered while telling all this in a soft voice.

"Janet, how did you cope with this horrendous situation?"

"How could anyone cope with this situation? I had to be strong for my kids' sake. For nearly two weeks this kind of begging and pleading for pain pills went on. Finally he died, much to my relief. I was strong for my kids. I went on with my life, raised my two boys by myself."

"Did you grieve?"

"No. I wanted to be strong for my kids. I just picked up the pieces and moved on. I had to go to work to pay my bills."

"You did not remarry."

"No. I had gone through enough with Ronny. He was a good man, but when he drank, he was mean. I did not want to go through another round of it. I could not risk exposing my kids to another man. You never know how that might affect them."

By now forty minutes had passed. Janet realized that we were getting close to the end of the interview, which she knew would last 50-60 minutes. She appeared much more relaxed than she was in the beginning of the interview, as I never once hassled her over her drug abuse issue.

"Well, doctor, like I told you there is nothing wrong with me or my life right now for me to suffer from this pain. I am not imagining this pain. What do you think is the cause of my pain?"

"You see, Janet, when you heard your son pleading for pain medications in exactly the same words as your husband did 22 years ago, all the buried painful emotions related to your husband's death surged-up like fizz coming up when a soda bottle is shaken-up vigorously. Since you believe in being strong, you had kept all those emotions buried in your hidden mind. Do you see how your pain resembles exactly the pain your husband suffered from? Your pain is the symbol of all that you went through with him 22 years ago."

Janet appeared to be stunned. She said that she had 'long forgotten' all that happened 22 years ago.

"You must have had some anger toward your husband for his drinking and dying on you like that, and also some guilt for enjoying the relief thereof. Did you?"

Janet nodded her head in agreement.

"I did. But I had two kids to raise and bills to pay. I had to put all this on the backburner and move on with my life."

"Janet, anger and guilt are two painful emotions, which prevent people from grieving when their loved one dies. So your emotional pain got buried in your hidden mind all these years. Two years ago, when you heard your son scream in pain exactly like your husband did 22 years before, it all came back up. Because you always coped with life by being strong, and you would not express your emotional pain, your body said, 'I will do the weeping for her.' Unexpressed painful emotions related to the dead person often result in people suffering from the same symptoms as the dead person."

Janet looked at me incredulously and said, "It seems farfetched to me. So this is all psychological, um? I am not imagining this, doctor."

"Well, Janet, I believe that your pain is real and your suffering is also real. Most people, including doctors, don't know that the mind and body are two interconnected parts of one single unit. What we think and how we feel affect every single organ in the body. And when the mind suffers, the body suffers with it. A vast network of nerves and circulating hormones connect these two seemingly different entities. If you bury your emotional pain in your hidden mind, it will come up sooner or later triggered by a similar later event. That results in serious symptoms."

"What should I do now?" asked Janet.

"If you get into counseling with a competent therapist and work through your anger, guilt and grief, your pain would gradually diminish and you would feel better over several months. Don't expect any quick fix."

"I am not a fan of therapy. I don't want to talk to strangers about my problem. I need to think about what you said. I am not certain that this is all in my mind."

"Janet, I understand. Here is a book I wrote about all this. Take it home and read it. Give some thought to it. If you want to talk with me again, I am here for you. Keep an open mind. OK? It was nice meeting with you. Bye."

I never saw Janet again. However, her doctor told me that she stopped abusing pain medicines from then onwards. If this patient got into counseling with a skillful counselor, she could be completely cured of her pain in due course. However, it takes time for patients to accept the reality that the brain/mind/body is one single unit. Secondly, getting better means risking losing Social Security Disability benefits. Thirdly, she has to accept the reality that her 'medical wild goose chase' was all a waste of money. She would look like a fool for being taken for a ride by all these medical professionals who were totally in the dark about the brain/mind/body connection, or else they would have asked for a psychiatric consultation early on.

Very often the chronic symptoms of patients such as Janet do not go away no matter what due to the phenomenon called 'secondary gain.' By staying sick, patients stand to gain money from disability insurance, and sympathy from family members and friends. By getting well patients risk losing them both. So symptoms persist. The question is, "What was the patient's 'primary gain?' Well, when Janet buried her painful emotions 22 years earlier, she immediately gained freedom from her emotional pain. That enabled her to move on with her life as if nothing ever happened.

2. "There is a woman from Florida on line two," said my secretary Kim on the intercom. "She wants to know if you will see her."

"Put her on," I said.

"Hello, Dr. Kamath. My name is Mildred. I have a doctor friend in Cape Girardeau. He told me to call you. I am at the end of the rope. I have suffered from severe trigeminal neuralgia for several years. I have seen several neurologists and have undergone surgery for it at Mayo Clinic. Nothing has helped. I saw a psychiatrist at Mayo. He told me I was depressed and I have chronic pain syndrome. I am depressed, but it is because I am hurting all the time. Will you please see me?"

"Mildred, you live in Florida and I am in Missouri," I said. "Won't it be hard on you to come here all the way from Florida? Do you have any relatives in Cape Girardeau?"

"I have no relatives there. But I can stay in a motel for two nights. I just want your opinion about it."

"All right. I will see you for one interview and give you an opinion. Don't expect any quick fix, though."

"I won't," she said. "I just want to know what is going on."

I was quite surprised by the fact that Mildred voluntarily wanted a psychological explanation for her neuralgia.

Two weeks later Mildred showed up for her appointment with her very supportive husband. She was a 55 year-old white woman. Her curly blondish hair was somewhat disheveled. She was at once eager to know what was wrong with her, and yet scared to know it. I noted that no one forced her to see me.

"Mildred, why don't you start by telling me about your suffering with trigeminal neuralgia?"

"I started having this pain under my left eye five years ago. Initially it came and went. Gradually it became constant and severe. Sometimes it is worse than other times. When it hits me, the pain is unbearable. I have throbbing pain in the left eye and it tears a lot. My face swells. I have to press my hand against my left eye for slight relief. I have seen many Ear, Nose and Throat specialists, neurologists, neurosurgeons and psychiatrists. I have taken antidepressant and anti-seizure medications without any relief. One doctor injected alcohol and glycerol into the nerve. Another even cut the nerve as it comes out of hole under my left eye. Nothing has helped. I went to Mayo clinic. They said that in some cases the problem is due to swelling of a blood vessel in the brain, which damages the trigeminal nerve. They even recommended that I undergo micro-vascular decompression surgery. I was scared to undergo that surgery. They had me evaluated by a psychiatrist. He diagnosed me as suffering from chronic pain syndrome and depression. He put me on antidepressant medication. It did not help me at all. Now I am on the seizure medication carbamazepine. It has not helped much. I am here as a last resort."

Mildred was tearful during most of this monologue, pressing her left eye with a folded handkerchief. I acknowledged her pain by saying, "I can see that you have a lot of pain, and you have suffered a lot in the past five years." Mildred nodded tearfully.

I began the stealth interview by asking her about her family. Mildred revealed that she has been married to her loving and supportive husband for thirty years. She raised two children, a boy and a girl. She worked as a librarian in a mid-sized city in Florida for nearly twenty years before she was forced to go on disability four years ago.

Mildred was born in Michigan as the second of two children of her parents. Her father was of German extract, child of first generation immigrants. He worked at a local auto factory for over forty years before retiring. He was emotionally distant from Mildred while she was growing up. Whenever she tried to get close to him, he pushed her away both emotionally and physically. She distinctly remembered many instances during her childhood when she tried to sit on his lap and he pushed her away. In contrast, her mother was loving and kind.

As an adult, it became an obsession with Mildred to win over her father's affection but without much success. She always wondered what did she do wrong to deserve such indifference and dislike.

7 years ago her mother died. At the funeral, she tried to console her father, but he was not receptive to her overture. She was very hurt by his continued rejection. A year after her mother's death, her father was admitted to a nursing home in Iowa because he was too feeble to take care of himself independently. Mildred's brother from Iowa called her to inform where her father was. Mildred felt sad for her father. She sent her father get-well cards, but he did not acknowledge them. She called him on phone, and he behaved like he could not hear her. In frustration, she hung up each time.

Finally, five years ago, Mildred decided to visit her father, whom she had not seen since her mother's funeral. She flew to Iowa, checked into a local motel and went to see him the next day. At the nursing home she checked in at the nurse's station. The head nurse directed her to her father's room. Mildred took a bouquet of flowers with her to cheer up her father. As she entered the room, she saw her father, frail, sick and old, sitting on a wheelchair. Seeing him thus, she broke into tears.

Mildred rushed to her father saying, "Hi, daddy! So nice to see you!" As she kissed him on his forehead, a teardrop fell on her father's left cheek just under his left eye. At this, her father became enraged and yelled, "Enough! Enough! Stop slobbering all over me!" Grabbing Mildred by her shoulder he pushed her away. Then with his gown he wiped off her tear from his face, and looked away from her.

Mildred was totally crushed by her father's rude behavior and rejection. She went into a daze and left the room sobbing. She was angry as hell at her father. She returned to Florida a broken woman. A few days after returning to Florida Mildred developed pain under the left eye and began her *medical wild goose chase.* Two years passed before she heard from her brother that her father died in the nursing home. She neither cried nor attended his funeral.

As Mildred told me this story, she had no clue about the connection between her hateful father wiping her tear from his left cheek and the pain over her own left cheek. After listening to her poignant story empathically, I explained to Mildred the following:

"Mildred, I believe that a lot of your trigeminal pain has to do with your emotional pain related to your father's rejection. Your pain started five years ago shortly after you returned to Florida following the painful encounter with your father. You have not been the same since. Your pain has been ever worse since your father died three years ago. When he rubbed away your tear from his left cheek and shouted 'Enough! Enough! Stop slobbering all over me!' his rejection was so final. You were devastated. Your trigeminal pain symbolizes that pain."

Mildred was stunned by this seemingly simplistic explanation. She sat silently for a while looking away from me. Then she said, "Doctor Kamath, what has my emotional pain to do with swelling of blood vessel in my brain? I have hard time believing this."

"Well, Mildred, when we lose someone we love, we grieve. When we grieve, the blood vessels in the head swell with blood. That is why our face swells and eyes get red. By weeping, we throw out the salt and water from those swollen blood vessels and reduce the pressure in them. Invariably we feel better after we cry, and face returns to its original color. The Brain, the mind and the body are one single unit. So from time to time some thought or emotion related to your father triggers swelling of your blood vessels in an attempt to get rid of those tears of grief. This aggravates your trigeminal neuralgia.

"Where do I go from here, Doctor?"

"When you return to Florida, search for a good counselor and get into therapy. In therapy, talk about your anger, hurt, disappointment, sadness and other painful emotions related to your father. Don't deny them; don't rationalize them; don't make excuses for them. Just get in touch with your deep-rooted emotions going back to your childhood; become more aware of them; release them by crying, sobbing and sighing. You will be amazed how well you begin to feel in due course. You have a lot of crying to do. It might take several weeks or even months for you to feel a lot better. But I know you will get better. If you are not better in two months after you get into therapy, come back for another session. In the mean time read this book I have written for people like you. Call me any time if you have any question."

When Mildred left my office, she seemed to be in a daze. She left for Florida the next day. I never heard from her again.

CHAPTER 5

Loss, Grief, Murder and Suicide

GRIEF IN REACTION TO A loss is fundamental to human condition. Throughout our life we experience loss of living beings we are emotionally attached to: Grandparents, parents, siblings, relatives, friends, neighbors, national leaders, animals, plants…etc. In fact, we grieve even when we lose nonliving objects when we lose them: Money, house, car and the like, and even when we lose intangible objects such as power, title, fame, and the like.

The vast majority of patients I treated in my office had been through a series of losses, which they had not coped with appropriately. By the time they came to see me, their psychic apparatus had broken down, or about to break down under the weight of grief, and they had come down with serious emotional disorder such as depression or anxiety.

Unfinished grief: This was the basis of a large number of depressed people I treated. They had lost some one dear, but were unable to grieve because feelings of guilt and anger blocked the flow of emotions. Here are two cases of unfinished grief, showing up as major depression:

1. Karen, a 43-year old single woman, a nurse in one of the local hospitals, came to see me for complaints of depression of three months duration. She said, "Ever since my older sister died, I have been feeling sad almost all the time. I can't concentrate in my work. I have made many mistakes at work. I wake up around 3 in the morning, and feel tired all day long. My appetite is not good. I have lost interest in things I used to enjoy, such as reading novels, playing tennis, watching movies, and the like. I saw a psychologist twice. We wasted our time arguing over some trivial thing."

Karen's background revealed that when she was 14 year old her mother died of cancer of breast. Karen revealed that she had an older sister to whom she was very close, who suffered from a severe case Rheumatoid arthritis.[11] Prior to dying from complications thereof, Karen's sister suffered pain and debilitation for many years. Since Karen lived over 100 miles away from her sister, and being employed as a nurse, she was not able to visit her sister as often as she wanted to. Karen confessed that when she did visit her sister, she returned home feeling depressed because she felt so

---

11 Rheumatoid arthritis is an autoimmune disease. Strong psychological factors are suspected to contribute to it.

helpless to do anything about her sickness. Her sister did not want to move to Cape Girardeau.

Then four months before her visit with me, Karen came to know that her sister died at home with no one by her side. Karen attended her sister's funeral, but was not able to cry. Within a month after this incident, she began to notice that she woke up at 3 a.m. The rest of the depressive symptoms began to appear one after another: crying spells, loss of appetite, tiredness, poor concentration, loss of interest in her usual hobbies and activities, feelings of hopelessness, etc. Now Karen was functioning at 50% of her usual capacity. She said, "I feel like a discharged battery of a car. I have starting trouble."

"Karen, how did you feel when you came to know that your sister had died?" I asked.

"I felt so sad, so, so, sad. She was hardly three years older than me. She suffered a lot, you know. I felt so bad that I was not there for her during her last days. I was so busy with my work. I just could not take off. I feel very bad."

Karen was now in tears. I offered her some tissue paper.

"I don't know how I could kick this funk I am in. Maybe I need some antidepressant drugs."

"Maybe, maybe not. Let us see. Karen, where is your sister buried?"

"In St. Louis."

"Have you visited your sister's grave since she was buried there?"

"No. I somehow can't push myself to go there."

"You seem to feel so guilty for not being there for her."

"Yes. I feel so guilty. She was the only sibling I had. She had no one to look after her. She died such as lonely death. I should have been there for her."

Karen went on to express much guilt for not being there for her sister.

"Do I need antidepressant medication to get over this depression?" Karen asked.

"Karen, you do have all the symptoms of a major depressive disorder," I said. "And you could benefit from a course of antidepressant medication. However, the drug merely covers-up your symptoms and gives you false sense of wellbeing. If you don't want to be depressed again, you need to finish your grief. Now that you have become aware of your feeling of guilt, it should be much easier for you to complete the grieving process. Once the grieving is completed, your depression should go away."

"Where do I go from here?"

"I want you to write a long letter to your sister. Take many days to complete the letter. It is hard, but being an intelligent woman you can do it. In that letter, express your guilt feelings and ask for your sister's forgiveness. When you have finished writing the letter, you will find it easier to visit your sister's grave. Go there. Read your letter to your sister. Grieve. Keep the letter on her grave. If possible, repeat this exercise several times. Also, remember your mother and grieve over her loss. I expect you to feel better within a month. If you want I will see you for a few sessions between now and then. If you don't feel better on your homework, come back for another session. We will figure out why you did not get better. Here is my card. Call me any time day or night."

Karen was pleasantly surprised to know she did not need to be on an antidepressant drug. She was even more surprised to know that I did not make another appointment for her. I never heard from Karen again. I was certain that she would have called me if she had not improved, for, we had made emotional connection.

2. Cathy was a 48-year old white woman who came to see me for depression of two years duration. Her depressive bout began immediately after her 15-year old only daughter and child died suddenly due to an acute respiratory distress syndrome (ARDS). She gave the following story about her daughter.

Kimberly was a beautiful girl, a sophomore in high school. She was in the school cheerleading group, and part of many extracurricular activities. Being the only child her parents doted on her. One day two years ago, she woke up in the middle of the night and told her parents that she was extremely short of breath. Her mother rushed her to the emergency room (E.R.) of the local hospital. The E.R. doctor examined her, did chest X-ray, and told Cathy, "She has flu. Here is some antihistamine prescription. Take it as directed. Follow-up with her pediatrician."

Cathy took Kim home. Within two hours, Kim was struggling to breathe. Cathy rushed her back to the E.R. 20 miles away. By the time she reached the hospital, Kim was unconscious. The E.R. doctor diagnosed her as ARDS, and arranged for her to be flown to St. Louis by helicopter. Kim died on way to St. Louis. Cathy was inconsolable.

After being in a state of deep depression for a few months, Cathy saw two counselors in succession. Even after several sessions she did not improve. Her family doctor put her on an antidepressant drug. This drug did not help her depression. Finally, as advised by a close friend, Cathy made an appointment with me.

After getting to know Cathy, I asked her if the two counselors she saw earlier asked her about her guilt and anger related to her daughter's tragic death. They did not. Cathy ventilated her feelings of guilt for believing the doctor that Kim's problem was just common flu. She acknowledged her anger toward the doctor who was obviously ignorant of the seriousness of Kim's lung problem, and also anger toward herself for not doing enough to save her daughter.

I asked Cathy if she had a medical degree. She said, "No."

"How could you have second guessed the doctor when he told you that Kim had a simple case of flu?"

"I could not."

"Then your guilt over the tragic death of Kim is irrational, isn't it?"

"I guess."

"It was the doctor's incompetence that caused your daughter's death isn't it?"

"Yes. But I have hard time getting angry at the doctor."

"Cathy, it is perfectly all right for you to feel anger toward the doctor. Being the E.R. doctor, he should have known about ARDS. Right?"

Cathy agreed with my reasoning.

"Guilt and anger often obstruct the flow of grief-related emotions. One must first express them before being able to complete the grieving process. This is no different from having to fish out wet clump of toilet tissue before flushing the toilet."

As she became more aware of her inner guilt and anger, Cathy went on to ventilate them in two more sessions. Her depression began to lift. I told her to visit her daughter's grave, continue to grieve and taper off of the antidepressant drug over the next few weeks. She agreed to make another appointment in a month if she did not feel better. I never heard from Cathy again.

Untreated at the early stage, patients such as Karen and Cathy would have become chronically depressed, and would have been on antidepressant drugs for many years to come.

Abandonment and its consequences: Childhood abandonment by parents, either by death or desertion, sensitizes people to abandonment later in life, resulting in intolerable emotional pain. Whereas more women attempt suicide, more men succeed in killing themselves. Some men commit murder as well as suicide. Here are three case studies:

1. Gary, a 47-year old *former patient* of mine came to my office around 1 p.m. with a loaded gun determined to assassinate me. I cannot explain why I was not in my office that afternoon, for I was always in my office at that time. My office manager Kim was alone in the office, typing a psychiatric report.

"Where is Dr. Kamath?" Gary asked Kim. Kim looked up from her typewriter and said casually, "I don't know. He is not here yet."

"When is he expected?" Gary asked gruffly.

"I have no idea. He should have been here already. Can I take a message?"

"No. I will be back a little later." Gary left the office and drove off.

An hour later, Gary was back in my office, more determined than ever to murder me. Not knowing his intention, my secretary told him that I had not returned to the office as yet and that she did not know when I would return. Frustrated, Gary drove off from my office parking lot.

When I returned to my office around 2 p. m., Kim told me that Gary had stopped by twice asking for me. I wondered why. I had terminated Gary from my care about six months earlier.

"What did he want? I asked.

"I don't know. I asked him, but he did not tell me."

I went home around 4.30 p. m. While having my dinner, I turned the television on to KFVS TV. To my horror, Gary was on the Breaking News.

After leaving my office, Gary headed in the direction of Sikeston, Missouri, 30 miles to the south where he lived. He pulled his pickup truck into the parking lot of the office of Dr. F., a local Ear, Nose and Throat (E.N.T.) specialist. He knew this doctor well, as they both attended the same church. Apparently Dr. F. had referred Gary to a psychiatrist in St. Louis, Missouri, shortly after I terminated him from my practice six months earlier.

Gary entered Dr. F.'s office and told the receptionist to tell Dr. F. to meet him in the parking lot. Not knowing what was going to happen, the good doctor showed up in the parking lot and asked, "Hi, Gary! What is going on?" Gary took out his loaded Smith and Wesson handgun from his pocket and pumped five bullets into the doctor's chest. He drove off immediately from there. The innocent middle-aged doctor, father of six children, was rushed to the local hospital where he died on the operating table. Gary drove straight to his fiancée's home a couple of miles away, shot her to death and then shot himself in the chest. When the SWAT team broke into the house, Gary was already dead.

One could only imagine the consequences of this great tragedy on the doctor's family as well as his staff who witnessed this tragedy, not to mention Gary's only son and other family members. Here is the background information on this case study:

Gary had been my patient since I opened my practice in 1982 for a simple case of chronic major depression, which was rooted in his childhood issues of *abuse* and *abandonment* by his parents. He had little motivation to get into therapy to deal with these deeply buried traumatic issues. He was quite satisfied with taking 200mg of an ancient "tricyclic" antidepressant medication known as amitriptyline to control his depressive symptoms. This medication helped him to be a functional human being. He worked for Missouri Department of Transportation.

When newer drugs known as "serotonergic" came into the market around 1990, he decided not to shift to one of them based on his belief, 'If it ain't broke don't try to fix it.' In addition to amitriptyline, Gary took 200mg of a useless and relatively harmless and inexpensive antidepressant drug called trazodone only to help him sleep better at night. Trazodone had little side effect except sedation.

Gary saw me for 15 minutes every six months for medication check. During the visit I asked him questions related to his medication and his mental health. He never paid his very small office fee as required before leaving my office. He sent me a check once in a while. When I asked him why he was not paying his bills at the time of his office visits, he always replied, "You will get paid. Don't worry." At any given time, he owed me fees for six office visits. As I always sensed a controlled rage in him, I chose not to antagonize him over this issue. Obviously he had transferred on to me his anger and disappointment with his own parents.

About eight months before the tragic incident, when I was vacationing abroad, Gary's pharmacist accidentally gave him trazodone 100mg tablets instead of 50 mg tablets. Gary took 4 tablets of 100mg that night thinking that he was taking 4 tablets of 50mg each. He woke up two hour later than his usual time of 6 a.m. He was late for his work. His 14-year-old son had already left for school. Wondering why he had slept 2 hours longer, Gary checked his bottle. He realized that his pharmacist had given him 100mg tablets by mistake. He became very scared that he might have died due to overdose. "What if I had died and my son became an orphan like me?" he thought. Memories of his childhood abandonment by his parents resurfaced and flooded his mind. Suddenly he experienced a massive panic attack. He started sweating profusely, his heart began to thump furiously, he felt pressure in his chest, he could hardly breathe, and he thought he was going to faint or die. He ran to the emergency room (E.R.) where he was checked thoroughly. The E.R. doctor told him that there was nothing wrong with him. The E.R. doctor assured him that no one had ever died from trazodone overdose. After staying in the hospital overnight, he went home.

A few days after I returned from my vacation, Gary came to see me. During his office visit he related to me the 'overdose' incident and said, "What bothered me the most was what if I had died and my son was made an orphan?" Gary had the sole custody of his son since his divorce from his boy's mother a few years earlier. Obviously Gary's own abandonment by his father when he was a boy was the issue at play here. Gary wanted to sue the pharmacist for damages even after the pharmacist apologized for his mistake and agreed to pay his medical bills. It was obvious that he was blaming the pharmacist for bringing up the buried abandonment issue. Gary asked me to give him a certificate that he incurred 'irreparable and permanent damage' to his body and mind due to the pharmacist's negligence. He was going to file a lawsuit against the pharmacist.

I reassured Gary that he suffered no permanent damage due to the accidental overdose. I told him that there were no reported cases of death or damage from overdose of trazodone. I had personally seen cases of overdose with 2000mg of trazodone, and none had died or suffered permanent damage to any body organ. Gary was not satisfied by this reassurance. He was out to avenge the pharmacist for his negligence. He insisted that I issue him a false certificate. When I politely declined, he left my office in a huff. Now a stage was set for adversarial relationship between Gary and myself.

Gary returned a few days later saying that he was very depressed and I should treat him for it. Now he was blaming me for his state of mind. He appeared rather angry with me. I reasoned with him that he needed to deal with his anger before adding any drugs, as his depression was worse because he was angry and disappointed that I did not issue him the certificate he wanted, and also due to resurfacing old traumatic memories. He must have felt abandoned by me as well. He denied being angry with me, and he refused therapy sessions. It was obvious that Gary was 'acting out' his anger. This left me with only one option: adding lithium to amitriptyline to 'augment' that drug. Gary refused lithium. It was clear that he was preparing the ground to punish me for my principled stand. Once again Gary left my office displaying much anger. As usual, he did not pay his bill.

Shortly thereafter I received a letter from a prominent local lawyer threatening to report me to the Board of Healing Arts for "unethical behavior." I wrote back explaining the details of this case and told him that far from being unethical I was being extremely ethical in refusing to issue Gary as false certificate. He was free to report me to the Board if he still thought he had a case against me. I wrote to him that there had never been a single complaint against me with the Board, and he would have to face the consequences if his reckless action caused any damage to my reputation. At this, the lawyer dropped Gary as his client.

Gary returned to my office claiming that his depression had worsened since his lawyer abandoned him. It was clear that he blamed me for his lawyer abandoning him. I tried to make him verbalize his anger without much success. It was clear that he was now after my blood. I told him that since he had turned down every treatment I offered him, I had nothing else to offer him. After he left my office in a fit of anger, I sent Gary a 30-day notice of termination from my practice citing our adversarial doctor-patient relationship. This was one of handful of terminations of patients during my practice.

I lost touch with Gary after he was terminated from my practice. After his death I heard from other sources that Dr. F. referred Gary to a psychiatrist in St. Louis, Missouri, 100 miles to the north. This psychiatrist admitted Gary to the hospital for the treatment of depression, which by now had become aggravated due to the stress of the preceding year's events not to mention resurfacing of 'abandonment issues' from his childhood. I had no direct access to his medical records since he left my practice, but a lawyer who interviewed me regarding this case told me that at the hospital the treating doctor stopped amitriptyline abruptly and started him on Fluoxetine. If this were true, that explained why Gary's condition went from bad to worse immediately. I had no way of assessing what went wrong with his treatment in St. Louis.

It is very likely that Gary blamed me for his unfortunate predicament. He must have thought that all his suffering would not have happened had I not refused him the certificate that trazodone overdose caused him irreparable damage. Since no court of law would side with him, he had no choice but to take the law into his own hands. Now he wanted me to pay for my "wrongdoing." Most likely he blamed Dr. F. for referring him to the doctor in St. Louis who, he must have thought, did him more harm than good. His rage was such that he had to kill somebody. He went home, loaded his handgun and came to my office to kill me. We may never know why he decided to kill his fiancée. It is possible that she threatened to abandon him, as she just could not handle his erratic behavior.

2. David, 48, a locksmith by profession, was admitted to the psychiatric ward for severe suicidal ideas. He said that his wife of two years was moving to St. Louis, 100 miles to the north. He just could not bear the separation. He tried to convince his wife to change her mind, but it was all in vain. He suspected that his wife was planning to divorce him. He has been traumatized by two previous divorces, and he was not going to go through another one. He would rather "blow my brains out" than suffer intolerable emotional pain.

A detailed history revealed that David lost his mother around age 7 from some unknown disease. His emotionally distant father and negligent stepmother raised him. At age 20 he got married for the first time. His wife could not deal with his clingy behavior rooted in his fear of abandonment. She left him within a year. David remarried five years later. His second wife also left him after two years. Again, he blamed himself for this divorce, as he believed that his controlling and clingy behavior was more than his wife could take. He did not get into therapy as he had low opinion about therapists. He remained single for many years, not daring even to date for fear of rejection.

About two years before his admission to the hospital, David met a beautiful woman during the course of his business as locksmith. Lori was very inviting and easygoing. David fell head-over-heels in love with her. He charmed her with a lot of attention, flowers and gifts. He wined and dined her and made her feel like a princess. Lori and David got married within two months of meeting. As if to compensate for all the deprivation of love he endured from his childhood, David began to cling on to Lori, and constantly demanded love and attention. He became extremely insecure and worried that other men might become attracted to her. He became increasingly controlling of her movements. Soon David was busy harassing her as to where she was, why she was late coming home, and the like. Within one year of the marriage, life became intolerably difficult for Lori. She began to spend more time at work just to get away from David. This only made David more insecure. His controlling behavior got worse.

Finally Lori decided to separate from David just to get some breathing room. Every time she mentioned separation, David flew into a rage. At times his behavior scared here. She then came up with the plan to get a job in St. Louis. That would give her the natural way out of this dysfunctional marriage. When David came to know about this plan, he panicked. He began to threaten suicide partly as manipulation to control Lori. However, by now she just had had it with David. She was ready to move on.

I met with Lori at the hospital in connection with David's treatment. Initially she insisted that she loved David and her move to St. Louis had nothing to do with David's clingy and controlling behavior. At this point I cut to the chase by saying, "Lori, would you believe a fish in the fisherman's basket, which claims it loves being there?" At this gentle confrontation Lori opened up and confessed to her feeling trapped in a marriage with a man traumatized by childhood abandonment. She just could not handle his controlling and harassing behavior arising from this issue. She wanted out.

In the ensuing marital therapy session, Lori expressed to David her unhappiness with his behavior, and her desire to move on with her life. When David promised to change, Lori said that her decision to leave him was final and nothing he said or did would change her mind. At this, David became very quiet. Lori left the meeting with tears in her eyes. David came across as stoic.

The next day David asked to be discharged from the hospital. He refused further therapy. When I told him that I was considering committing him involuntarily to a state hospital, he replied, "Doc, I can open any lock. I can walk away any time I want to. Do you think anyone could keep me from killing myself if I really wanted to? If you commit me to the state hospital, I will tell them that I have no desire to die. They will have to let me go." Since he was a voluntary patient, I had no choice but to let him go.

That evening I got a phone call from the hospital E.R. doctor. He said that an ambulance had just brought in David's body without his skull. When I went to the E.R., his dead body was on the gurney, with a few loose pieces of his skull. His brain had been totally blown off. Apparently David had held a Colt 45 to his right temple and blown his own brains out. I took solace in the fact that at least he had not killed Lori, like it happens once too often if people with abandonment issues. There was not anything anyone could do to save this man from himself. His past had finally caught up with him.

3. Robert, a 39-year old married farmer checked into the psychiatric ward complaining of severe depression. His wife said that over the past three months he often threatened to kill himself. Neither Robert nor his wife could tell me what happened recently that might have triggered Robert's suicidal depression.

Robert was born as one of two children of his parents who were farmers. He had a younger sister. While growing up, he was very close to his mother. His father was unfaithful to his mother, and he often witnessed his mother crying over it. When he was 8 years old his mother died in a car accident. Robert said he did not remember much about this tragic event. When asked if he felt any sadness over his mother's death, he said, "I don't remember anything about my mother."

Robert's father remarried a few years later, but Robert did not get along well with his stepmother. As an adolescent Robert was insecure in his relationship with girls he dated. Several girls broke up with him because of his clingy and controlling behavior. When he was 30 years old, he met a woman who became his wife. They raised two children. Now the boy was 8 and girl was 5 years old.

Robert said that about three months before his admission to the hospital, he saw a change in his wife's behavior towards him. She appeared to be emotionally distant from him, which upset him a lot. He said, "I just could not figure out what was going on." In his presence his wife denied she had become emotionally distant from him.

Suspecting the veracity of her statement, I met with Lois alone. She revealed that Robert had always been clingy and controlling during 9 years of their marriage, but over the past year he had been insufferably clingy. He would not let her out of his sight. If she came home late even by an hour, he gave her 'third degree.' As his behavior became more intolerable, she began to lose affection for him. She met a man at work who comforted her. One thing led to another and she got into an ongoing affair with the coworker. Lois wanted a divorce, but she could not tell Robert about it in the state of mind he was in. However, now that he was in the hospital under my care, she felt compelled to level with him and get it all over with.

I explained to Lois that the reason why Robert had been clingier and more controlling over the past few months was because their son was nearing the age of 8, the age at which he lost his mother in the car accident. The buried grief over his mother's death was resurfacing, causing Robert to fear losing her as well. He was re-experiencing his insecurity as an 8-year old child. Obviously, Robert did not want to let his wife out of sight for fear of losing her, without realizing that his behavior actually drove her away from him.

This explanation of Robert's behavior did not move Lois. She said that it was time for her to come clean with Robert. She asked me to help him to accept his loss and move on with his life. I agreed to meet with them both to facilitate the process. In the meeting, Lois told him that she had been feeling stifled in the relationship and that it was time they split up. Robert did not show any emotion. He asked Lois if she was having an affair. She admitted that she was. At this, Robert said, "I knew that something was going on, but I could not put my finger on it. Now that I know, I feel better. Now it is all in the open, and I need not torment myself. I feel better knowing the truth."

After Lois left the hospital, I met with Robert again to assess how he was doing. He appeared calm, and he said again that he felt better knowing Lois' affair. He said that he had checked into the hospital just to resolve this issue once and for all. Now that it is resolved, there was no reason for him to stay in the hospital any longer. He promised not to harm himself or his wife. Since he was a voluntary patient, and there was no evidence of imminent suicidal intent, I had no choice but to discharge him from the psychiatric ward. There was no evidence to legally commit him involuntarily to a State Hospital.

Three hours later Lois called me. Calmly she said,

"Dr. Kamath, Robert came home, loaded his rifle, and shot himself to death."

I was stunned. I should have known better. He was already under a great deal of stress due to resurfacing grief over his mother's death triggered by his son turning 8. Now knowing that his wife was having an affair and was going to abandon him pushed him over the brink. Robert must have felt that he just could not take it anymore.

Though this tragedy shook me up a great deal, I coped with it by resorting the reality that if someone was determined to end his life, psychiatrist could do little to prevent it.

CHAPTER 6

Emergency!

I OFTEN RECEIVED PHONE CALLS from the hospital and doctors asking me to attend to emergencies on the floor. Here are three cases studies among the hundreds I treated over three decades.

1. The chief nurse on the psychiatric ward called me frantically and said, "We are all very worried about Chandra, a 15-year old inpatient on the psychiatric ward. She stopped eating and drinking two days ago. She is now in bed in fetal position. She urinates and defecates in bed. She looks dehydrated. I think you need to see her right away. She might need to be on the medical floor with intravenous fluids or gastric tube."

David, the child psychologist who was treating Chandra, said he had seen her a couple of times in his office before admitting her to the psychiatric floor four days ago. She told him that she had suicidal thoughts. Following the admission to the ward, he saw Chandra everyday and she steadily regressed. When the chief nurse asked Chandra why she was not eating, she replied feebly, "I just want to go home." However, David did not want to discharge her because she had made suicidal threats.

I reviewed Chandra's chart and came to the conclusion that she was a victim of David's aggressive interrogation. Obviously, he was an inexperienced therapist. I had to rescue her from his care immediately. I asked the chief nurse to accompany me to Chandra's bed. Chandra looked very feeble, lying in fetal position in the bed. It was obvious that she had regressed to being a child. I pulled a chair and sat by the side of the bed and introduced myself to her. She did not open her eyes. I held Chandra's right hand gently and said, "Chandra, I am doctor Kamath. You want to go home, right?" Chandra nodded her head without opening her eyes. I said to her, "I will send you home right now if you agree to eat your breakfast and take a shower."

Chandra opened her eyes and looked at me incredulously. I could see by the look on the chief nurse's face that she was horrified by my decision to send her home right away in the state of mind and body she was in. I asked the nurse to fetch a glass of water. She did so promptly. I told Chandra to sit upright. Slowly she did as told. I held the glass to her mouth and she drank all of it. I then told the chief nurse, "Get her a plate of breakfast." I fed Chandra her breakfast a little at a time, and she ate all of it over the next fifteen minutes. She seemed to feel better rapidly.

Then I told Chandra, "You need to take a nice shower. Are you up to it?" She nodded her head. I asked the chief nurse to escort her to the bathroom and assist her in taking a good bath.

Fifteen minutes later Chandra was back in her bed, looking very different from what she was like a just 30 minutes earlier.

I told the chief nurse to get Chandra's discharge papers ready. When she left the room, I asked Chandra what happened to make her feel so upset. She replied that David had been badgering her to tell her why she was depressed. She said, "I don't know why I was depressed. He kept telling me that I was not being truthful. He would not let up. I just could not take it anymore." Escape from David's clutches improved her immediately.

The chief nurse returned with paperwork. I signed the order for discharge. I called Chandra's mother, a nurse in the Emergency Room, to come upstairs to the ward to take Chandra home. When she showed up at the ward, she was overjoyed to see the dramatic change in Chandra. She said, "When I saw her early this morning, I was truly worried about her. She looks like her normal self. What happened?"

"Well," I said, "sometimes therapists and hospitals do more harm than good. Need I say more?" Being a nurse herself, Chandra's mother nodded understandingly. I told the mother to make an appointment for Chandra with the experienced and compassionate female psychiatrist at the mental health center.

Several years later when I stepped into the elevator at the same hospital, I saw a pretty young woman smartly dressed in Navy uniform. Her face looked familiar. She smiled and I said, "Don't I know you?"

"I am Chandra," she said. "I can't thank you enough for saving my life!" She said that since her discharge from the hospital, she moved on with her life, finished high school and joined the Navy. She added, "I am doing great!"

This is a classic example of how therapy in the hands of inexperienced mental health professionals could do more harm than good. Very often patients become suicidal shortly after beginning therapy, and end up in the hospital. This is because inexperienced therapists bring up buried issues, which flood the patient's already overloaded mind and cause intolerable stress. It is as if their soda bottle is vigorously shaken and the fizz enters the balloon attached at the top, which is already full.

2. The nurse from the third floor of the local hospital was frantic. She said, "Dr. Kamath, please come over here quickly. This man is ready to jump out of the window. He has suddenly become psychotic. We have him on restraints. His doctor ordered Haldol. That did not help. Please hurry!"

When I entered the patient's room, I saw a middle-aged man in bed. His hands and feet had been tied down to the bed with leather straps. He was struggling to escape from his restraints. He kept shouting, "Let me go!" It was obvious that he was completely out of his mind.

"We had given him two shots of Haldol in the past hour," said the nurse. "It has not touched him a bit." Haldol is a powerful antipsychotic drug.

I asked the nurse to bring me the patient's chart. When I read his doctor's admission note, it said that he had been on carbamazepine (Tegretol), an anti-seizure medication for several years for an unspecified pain syndrome. When I looked at the patient's current medications, carbamazepine was not on the list. His doctor had stopped this drug three days earlier because he thought that the patient did not need it. Obviously, the patient's psychotic behavior was caused by carbamazepine withdrawal. Obviously, the treating neurologist did not know that drugs working on the brain should never be stopped abruptly.

"Get me four tablets of carbamazepine immediately," I told the nurse. She ran to the nurses' station and brought four tablets of the drug. I told the patient that he was having withdrawal from his drug and he needed to eat the pills immediately. He shook his head in agreement. I put four pills in his mouth and gave him a cup of water to wash them down. I assured him that he would be all right pretty soon. I then wrote in his chart that his regular dose of carbamazepine should be restarted immediately. I left the ward telling the nurse to contact me in one hour.

An hour later the ward nurse called me saying that the patient had calmed down considerably. I told her to release him from his restraints. When I visited the patient that evening, he was back to his normal self. Many years later this man approached me in a shopping center and thanked me for saving his life. As I had no recollection of this incident, he reminded me by saying, "If you had not restarted my Tegretol, I would have jumped out of the window."

I have lost count of emergencies I had seen such as this, mostly caused by discontinuation of drugs the patient had been taking for years because, "his attending doctor thought he did not need it." Usually, they stopped medications such as alprazolam (Xanax), Lorazepam (Ativan), amitriptyline, and the like. Most doctors don't seem to know that drugs that work on the brain should never be stopped abruptly. Even after I told many doctors never to do that, they kept repeating the same mistake. I was forced to conclude that it was far more difficult to educate doctors than patients.

While I am at it, let me recount here how abrupt withdrawal of a drug caused a family to break up. When examining a 40-year old female patient, a doctor saw bluish discoloration under her nails. He thought that this was due to a side effect of a beta-blocker drug propranolol (Inderal), which she had been taking for many years. The doctor panicked and told her to stop it immediately. He did not know that this drug enters the brain and calms it down. Immediately after stopping this short-acting drug, the patient became highly irritable, hostile and unbearably critical of her husband. Sometimes she became physically violent with him. Soon they were fighting over nothing. The husband did not know what to make of this sudden change in his wife's behavior. Over the next few weeks he lost his love for her. Within a couple of months, he told her that he wanted a divorce. By the time I saw them together, his feelings had hardened, and he no longer wanted to be married to her. They broke up and their children were traumatized by this unfortunate development caused by the doctor's ignorance of the drug he prescribed.

I have lost count of such horror stories in the course of my practice. Here one example of many I was called to see in the hospital. A patient was admitted to the hospital for severe urinary tract infection. History revealed that she developed a distended bladder shortly after her doctor prescribed her a psychotropic drug, which has the side effect of relaxing the bladder muscles. The doctor did not know about this side effect. So when the patient complained about inability to urinate, he asked a urologist to see her. He did a cystoscopy on the patient and put her on a drug to help the bladder contract. Soon the patient developed a severe urinary tract infection. She was hospitalized. Because her original psychiatric condition got aggravated, the doctor called a psychiatric consultation. So on and so forth. All this could have been avoided if the doctor knew the side effect of the psychotropic drug he prescribed, and gave the patient an antidote.

In fact, when patients asked their doctors if the drug they prescribed interacted with the one I prescribed, their standard reply was, "I don't know. Call Dr. Kamath. He knows his medicine better I." Invariably, when these patients called me, I gave them the needed information, but also asked them, "Do you feel safe when your doctor prescribes you a drug and tells you that he does not know its drug-drug reaction with the drug I prescribed?"

3. I got a phone call from Dr. Davis. He said, "Bob, I need your help right away. I have this young man in the Intensive Care Unit. He is withdrawing from alcohol. He is delirious. I have him in restraints. I have given him a lot of tranquillizers, but nothing has helped him. I would appreciate if you could see him right away."

Obviously, this young man was suffering from what is known as delirium tremens. This condition has very high mortality. Untreated, about 40% of these patients die.

I rushed the hospital I.C.U. The patient was a young man in full restraints. He was very agitated and hallucinating. The nurses had somehow kept his intravenous drip running. I reviewed his chart and noted that he had been given a large dose of a minor tranquillizer Librium. The main problem now, however, was that the patient had become psychotic. If he were continued to struggle while still in restraints, soon his muscles would breakdown and he would go into kidney failure. I must do something immediately.

I told the nurse to give the patient a shot of 5 mg of Haldol, a potent antipsychotic drug. Within ten minutes of the shot, the patient calmed down. I put the patient on Haldol 5 mg by mouth three times a day.

Just then Dr. Davis entered the I.C.U. He was incredulous at the improvement in the patient. He could not resist saying, "Bob, what kind of miracle is this?"

"This is no miracle, Dr. Davis," I said. "The guy had become psychotic. Minor tranquillizers don't work on psychosis. So I gave him a major tranquillizer to control his psychosis. We can taper off of this drug once he is stable."

Over the next 24 hour, the patient improved to the point that he was transferred to the general ward. He was discharged home in three days.

A few years later, when I was making rounds at a local nursing home, a young man, working there as nurses aide, approached me. "Hi Dr. Kamath," he said. "Do you recognize me?"

"I am sorry, I don't," I said.

"You saved my life," he said. "Some years ago I was in the I.C.U. having delirium. Dr. Davis was at the end of the rope."

"Oh, yes!" I said. "I remember now. You look good!"

"I stopped drinking after that horrible incident. That scared the hell out of me. I have been clean ever since. "

CHAPTER 7

What My Patients Taught Me

CAREFULLY LISTENING TO THOUSANDS OF people I evaluated for various agencies and patients I treated in my 40-year long medical practice taught me the information I have given in this chapter. It gives readers a general outline of stress and various stress-related issues we discussed in the previous chapters.

IS STRESS CONTAGIOUS?

Yes, stress is contagious. There is much truth in the following story: An irate woman verbally abuses her timid husband, a schoolteacher. Humiliated, the teacher takes his anger out on his student by paddling him. Outraged over the unjust punishment, the student kicks his hapless dog. The resentful dog bites the lazily snoozing cat. The incensed cat works out its frustration by mauling an unlucky rat. Running scared for its life, the wounded rat topples an oil lamp, shattering it into a thousand pieces on

painful emotions in response to upsetting situations. Thirty-six of them are responsible for bringing on many stress symptoms and disorders:

> *Fear, hurt, anger, sadness, guilt, shame, disappointment, frustration, helplessness, hopelessness, humiliation, hate, bitterness, resentment, envy, jealousy, terror, horror, disgust, embarrassment, rage, exasperation, insecurity, despair, dejection, remorse, regret, worthlessness, hostility, vengefulness, dread, sorrow, sinfulness, despondency, uselessness and powerlessness.*

The presence of these potentially toxic, painful emotions in the brain causes the brain chemicals to change, resulting in the appearance of *stress symptoms.* In other words, *pain in the brain* is the basis of stress symptoms. The brain is connected to the body organs via circulating hormones and a vast network of nerves. Changes in brain chemicals are felt as changes in the *functions* of the body organs, such as the heart, lungs, stomach and skin. Stress symptoms are the brain's way of warning us: *"I am sensing many toxic, painful emotions in your mind. Get rid of them as soon as possible or do something to stop them from coming in."* This is no different from a fire alarm going off when it detects more than the usual amount of smoke in the room.

Therefore, accepting the fundamental fact that the brain/mind/body is one single unit, and that emotions we experience affect every single organ in the body, is essential in understanding the phenomenon of stress and stress-related disorder.

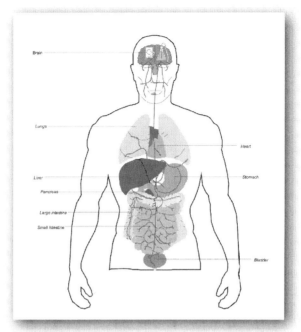

Picture#4: Brain/Mind/Body is one single unit

The brain is *hardwired* to produce different groups of stress symptoms in response to different painful emotions. For example, *fear* and its cohorts in the brain produce a "fight or flight" response; *sadness* and related emotions produce stress symptoms related to "grief"; *anger* and allied emotions produce an "attack" type of stress response such as irritability, hostility, rage; and *guilt* and related emotions produce "guilty" behavioral responses such a remorse. Readers interested in mastering the art of coping with stress must thoroughly learn about the nature of painful emotions, how they produce different stress symptoms and how to handle them. In other words, one must become *emotionally savvy if one wishes to cope with and manage stress.* In coping with stress, one's Emotional Quotient (EQ) is more important than one's Intelligence Quotient (IQ). I have met many highly intelligent people who had very low EQ. Not only were they unaware of their inner emotions, but also they lacked the ability to experience empathy for other people's emotional pain.

STRESSOR IS AN EVENT OR A PROBLEM THAT UPSETS US

A. Sensory input. Our conscious mind is constantly bombarded with information from the world around us. The five senses— seeing, hearing, touch, smell and taste—are conveyor belts that bring thousands of bits of information into the conscious mind/ balloon on a daily basis. This continuous inflow of information is known as *sensory input.* The nature of most of the incoming information is *neutral*; that is, we feel neither good nor bad about it. For example, if you look at a chair, you feel neither good nor bad about that chair, unless someone had hit you on the head with that chair. Some of the incoming information is perceived by our mind as *good*, and we feel happy about it. For example, if you get a phone call from your boss telling you that he is pleased with your performance and that he is giving you a big raise, you would feel happy. Some other information is perceived by our mind as *bad* for us. For example, if you were told that your performance at work was not good and you could be fired from your job at any time, you would feel very upset. Any event or problem that upsets us is known as a *stressor.*

B. Two types of stressors: Basically, there are two types of stressors: bad events and bad problems. Often bad problems follow bad events, and contribute to one's sickness.

1. **One-shot bad events**—such as the death of a loved one, the breakup of a relationship, betrayal or infidelity, an accident, robbery, assault, rape, the loss of a job, etc.— are extremely upsetting. They are *one-shot* painful events. When bad events occur, we experience many painful emotions in our conscious minds all at once, such as fear, terror, hurt, anger, sadness, guilt, shame and disappointment. The mind/balloon inflates suddenly with these painful emotions, and we experience severe stress symptoms. We refer to this kind of stress as *acute stress.*

Very often, bad events are the cause of bad problems. For example, death of a child could lead to divorce of parents. Loss of job could lead to serious financial problem. In people suffering from serious emotional disorders, we often find both these issues fueling their sickness.

2. **Bad problems** of life—such as problems with one's job, money, health, relationships, etc.—are *ongoing* life problems. They upset us a little bit at a time, day after day, week after week and month after month. Often, we *feel trapped* in these bad problems. In this case, the mind/

balloon inflates gradually, over a period of time, with painful emotions such as anger, fear, bitterness, resentment, insecurity, frustration or helplessness, and the stress symptoms are not as dramatic as when they are caused by a single bad event. If unsolved, most bad problems lead to the balloon popping because of the relentless buildup of painful emotions in the mind. When the balloon pops, one is brought down with a serious stress disorder, such as major depression or panic disorder. This type of stress is known as *chronic stress.*

C. The bicycle pump is an ideal model for stressors: Since bad events and life problems *pump painful emotions* into the conscious mind/balloon, let us represent them by a simple bicycle pump. Bad events and bad life problems have something else in common with the pump: *they both suck!*

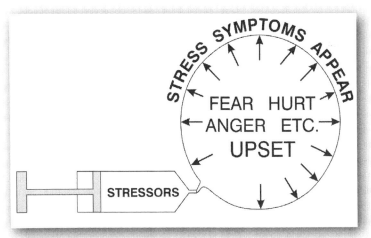

Picture 5: Stressors pump painful emotions into the mind.

THE HIDDEN MIND

How does the conscious mind decide what is bad for it? The mind has a hidden compartment, like the basement of a house or the hard drive of a computer, where it had stored a large amount of information that was gathered over a lifetime. The information pertains to whether an object or situation is good or bad for the mind: if it is bad, how bad, as well as how to react to it. As the powerful hard drive of a computer saves millions of bits of information in its numerous folders and files, this hidden compartment of the mind holds millions of bits of information in its folders and files. Every time the conscious mind receives some input from one or more of the five senses, it checks with the hidden mind, "What is this? Is it good or bad for me? If it is bad, how do I react to it?" For example, if a stranger offered you a cookie, your conscious mind would ask your hidden mind, *"Is this safe to eat?"* Your hidden mind might say something such as, *"You don't know this person. The cookie he's offered could be dangerous. Don't eat it."* This type of interaction takes place between the conscious mind and the hidden mind thousands of times a day. If your hidden mind does not know whether something is good or bad for you, your conscious mind would feel baffled or confused. A person whose hidden mind does not have the information needed to make the right decision in response to a piece of sensory input is said to be *naïve,* or innocent. Therefore, they exercise poor judgment in assessing the danger of a situation. We warn our naïve children about the dangers of the world by saying such things as *"Don't talk to strangers! Don't accept cookies from strangers! Don't get into the car with strangers!"* In other words, we pass on to our children the wisdom we had gained from our past experience.

The soda bottle is an ideal model for the hidden mind: We can compare the hidden mind to a soda bottle filled with gaseous soda. Just as the dissolved gas in the soda is invisible until the bottle is shaken, all the information in the hidden mind is *out of our immediate awareness* until some sensory input activates it and brings it to our awareness. For example, right now, you are not thinking of Donald Trump—until you read his name here. Immediately after reading it, your conscious mind might see his image on the screen of your mind, and you might experience neutral, good or bad emotions related to him. If you are a Republican you would feel good about him. If you were a Democrat, you would feel bad about him. After a while, his image will disappear from the screen and go back into the "Memory Folder" of your hidden mind.

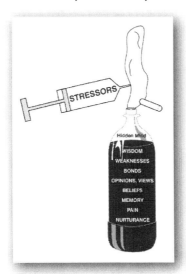

Picture 6: The hidden mind holds millions of bits of information in its folders.

Coping simply means shrinking the balloon

Coping with stress simply means being able to shrink the balloon by *appropriate methods*. This action gets rid of the toxic, painful emotions from the mind, and allows the brain chemicals to go back to their original position. Then the stress symptoms disappear. Coping requires us to become *aware* of the painful emotions in the conscious mind; get rid of them by *expressing* them; *cancel them out* by means of various mental skills such as putting things in proper perspective, changing perception, cancelling out painful emotion by means of opposite emotions, and many other methods.

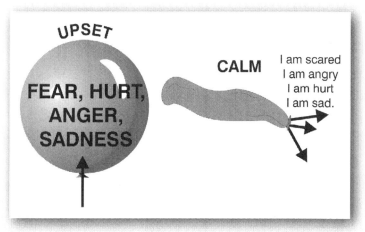

Picture#7: Expressing painful emotions makes symptoms disappear

Often the grieving process is hindered by guilt and anger. Therefore, for one to express grief, one must first get rid of these two emotions.

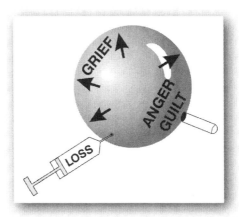

Picture 8: Anger and guilt often block expression of grief

Coping with stress also requires us to skillfully turn off the pump by *solving the problems* that are hounding us. In other words, we need to pull the plug on the pump. Then we calm down, and peace and tranquility return to the mind.

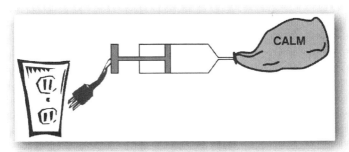

Picture#9: Solving problems makes stress symptoms go away

It's as simple as that—except that stressed-out people are not able to do any of these things. That is why they need a shrink to do the shrinking for them, and to educate them about appropriate coping methods. Unfortunately, most psychiatrists these days attempt to control the symptoms of depression and anxiety by coating the balloon with drugs, rather than by shrinking it or teaching people how to shrink it themselves.

Let us represent coping mechanism by a tube coming out of the right side of the balloon (see picture 10). Now the model of the mind is complete.

The completed model of the mind

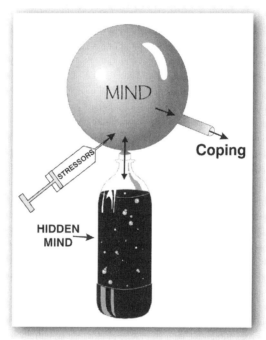

Picture #10: The model of the mind.

Let us briefly review the completed model of the mind as shown above. The bicycle pump in the picture above represents stressors. As soon as the conscious mind/balloon receives sensory input from the pump, it asks the hidden mind (soda bottle) about the nature of this input. When told, "This is bad," the conscious mind becomes upset. The balloon inflates with painful emotions such as fear, hurt, anger, sadness, etc.; the brain chemicals change and stress symptoms appear, as shown in picture#3. The side tube represents those actions that shrink the balloon, such as expressing emotions and solving problems.

For example, if someone we love dies, the balloon would immediately inflate with painful emotions related to grief: sadness, hurt and sorrow. Inflation of the balloon will cause the appearance of severe stress symptoms: fullness in the chest, swelling of the face, intensely sad feelings. By grieving, crying, sobbing and expressing our emotions (using the side tube), we shrink the balloon and get rid of stress symptoms. Those who are able to keep the balloon shrunk all the time stay well.

The main idea of coping is that the *output of painful emotions should equal the input.* The reader must thoroughly understand this model of the mind and the interaction between its four components if he/she wants to learn about stress.

MANAGING STRESS MEANS LEADING A WISDOM-BASED LIFESTYLE

Whereas coping has to do with ridding the conscious mind of painful emotions *after* one has become upset, managing stress has to do with *preventing* upsetting events and problems from happening.

Managing stress simply means living a lifestyle that minimizes the occurrence of bad events and problems. This boils down to making *wise choices* in all aspects of life. To accomplish this, we have to wisely manage our relationships, money, time, health, job and other aspects of daily life. The bottom line in stress management is that one should live a simple life guided by wisdom. This raises the question: What is wisdom?

There is some truth in the saying that wisdom comes from experience and experience comes from stupidity. We learn from mistakes we made due to our lack of knowledge about the world. The adage that those who do not learn from their mistakes are condemned to repeat them is very true. Wisdom is the sum total of the following seven basic elements: Knowledge about the world at large; memory of lessons learned from mistakes we made and life experiences; judgment about people and situations in life; ability to reason when presented with facts; ability to develop insight into one's own mind; moral values based on time-honored 'thou shall not' proscriptions, and finally noble virtues, such as compassion, generosity, altruism, love for humanity, opposition to injustice, and many other such attributes.

A wise person always *does the right thing*. For example, to avoid money problems, he lives within his means, saves money regularly, refrains from incurring nonessential debts, does not get into businesses about which he knows nothing, etc. To avoid health problems, he resists bad habits, gets adequate exercise, and takes good care of his body. To avoid conflicts with others, he holds back from imposing his views on people or taking advantage of their friendships; he engages others in adult to adult interactions, and so on. In effect, stress management means gaining a good deal of control over all aspects of one's life (the pump).

Stress management also requires that we *avoid making wrong choices* and doing wrong things. Both these mistakes are always based on deep-rooted *personality weaknesses,* such as greed, hatred, possessiveness, arrogance, jealousy, stinginess, insecurity and prejudice. One or more of these personality weaknesses, fuel every serious life problem, whether it is connected to one's job, money, health, relationship or law. Religious texts such as the Bible teach people the importance of leashing these evil qualities to prevent serious life problems. Unfortunately, many people's focus is on practicing the mindless rituals of their religion than on applying the morals the good book recommends. I have lost count of crooked businessmen I had come across, who said they were Sunday school teachers and never missed a single Sunday church service. Here is a classic example:

A middle-aged married man came to see me for complaints of severe anxiety. His history revealed that he was a drug addict as well as drug supplier. A son was in jail on drug charges when he committed suicide. The patient said he supplied street drugs to members of his church. He said that his profession was such that he had free access to the houses of his church members. He claimed that he was a staunch Christian, and Sunday school teacher.

It became evident that he was in my office to get a prescription for addictive tranquilizers. He had no awareness that his son's suicide had something to do with his evil lifestyle. When I tried to raise his awareness, he became very upset. The next day he called me and cursed me with every crude word he had learned on the streets. I listened to him patiently and thanked him for the call. I sent him back the fee he had paid me the day before with a note: "May Jesus give you the wisdom to do the right thing from now onwards." I wanted to teach him the true meaning of Mathew: 5:39: *But I say unto you, That ye resist not evil: but whosoever shall smite thee on thy right cheek, turn to him the other also.*

HOW DOES STRESS LEAD TO STRESS DISORDERS?

To most depressed or anxious patients, why they suffer from these maladies is a great mystery. They go to their doctors with symptoms such as sleeplessness, anxiety, mental and physical tension, crying spells, tiredness, poor concentration, etc. After thoroughly examining and testing them, the doctors tell them that no medical reason could be found for their seemingly serious symptoms. To make sense of the symptoms, the doctors then tell them that the disorder is a result of a *chemical imbalance.* However, the truth is that the chemical imbalance is the end result of an extraordinary amount of stress combined with poor coping.

Reading this, almost all people in such a situation might wonder, *"How could this be when I handled my stress so well by being strong?"* Therein lies the problem. People who readily fall apart when upset never become sick with stress disorders. And curiously, by the time a person is down with a stress disorder, he/she has *blocked off* from his awareness almost all his painful emotions, as well as the memory of stressful events and the problems that caused them.

A. History of serious traumas: The symptoms of the stressed-out person are just the tip of the iceberg (see picture 11 below). Every person suffering from stress disorder has been through many bad events and problems in his life, and he has experienced numerous painful, toxic emotions related to these bad events and problems. His balloon has inflated many times because of death of loved ones, abandonment, betrayal of trust, conflict, disappointment, assault, accident, physical, emotion and sexual abuse, breakups, serious illness and other tragedies. Bad memories of these events and problems, stored in his hidden mind, have become the submerged part of the iceberg.

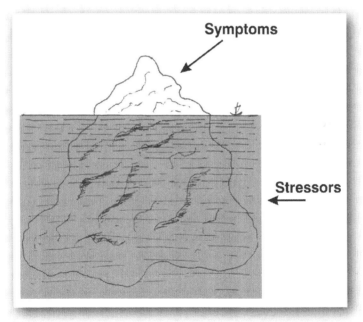

Picture# 11: Stress symptoms are just the tip of the iceberg.

B. A stressed-out person has had an overdose of painful emotions: In response to these serious bad events and problems of life, the stressed-out person has repeatedly experienced large doses of toxic, painful emotions in his mind, such as the thirty-six painful emotions we noted earlier. The majority of stressed-out people admit to empathic therapists having experienced most, if not all, of these painful emotions in large doses, over several years prior to becoming sick. In fact, most of them are surprised to know that they had harbored those painful emotions in their mind.

C. Coping by burying: As painful emotions flood the conscious mind, the stressed person gets rid of them, shrinks his balloon and calms himself down by making *one simple mistake:* instead of shrinking his balloon by expressing them and solving the problem, he says to himself, *"This is too upsetting for me. I will be strong. I will not think about it, I will not talk about it, I will just forget it."* He simply puts the painful emotions out of his awareness by burying them in his hidden mind/soda bottle. In other words, he *bottles up* his emotions. The balloon shrinks; the brain chemicals go back to their normal state and the stress symptoms disappear. The prompt relief from stress symptoms fools the person into believing that he *handled* his stress well, and that gives him a false sense of security. Since this method of burying (hiding or bottling up) painful emotions in the hidden mind seems to work well, it becomes a habit. However, all that this person is doing is transferring his painful emotions from the conscious mind/balloon to the hidden mind/soda bottle (see picture 12).

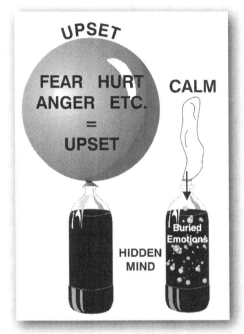

Picture# 12: Burying causes the balloon to shrink,
and makes the person feel calm once again.

D. The saturation point of the hidden mind: The problem
is that the hidden mind *does not have a limitless capacity* to store
painful emotions, just as the computer hard drive does not have
limitless capacity to store information, or the basement of a house
does not have limitless capacity to store garbage. As the person's
hidden mind (soda bottle) keeps filling up with painful emotions,
he finds it harder and harder to calm himself down by burying
them. When the hidden mind finally reaches its *saturation point,*
he can no longer bury his painful emotions. Now, when painful

emotions related to new bad events and problems appear in the conscious mind/balloon, they stay there. The re-inflated balloon responds by obeying Rule #1: When the balloon inflates, stress symptoms appear.

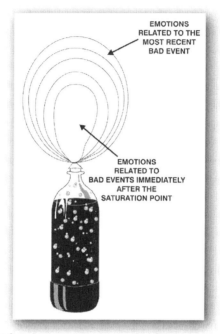

EMOTIONS
RELATED TO THE
MOST RECENT
BAD EVENT

EMOTIONS
RELATED TO
BAD EVENTS IMMEDIATELY
AFTER THE
SATURATION POINT

Picture# 13: After the saturation point the balloon starts to re-inflate.

As the balloon gets bigger and bigger, more stress symptoms begin to reappear one by one, become persistent and get worse over time. As more painful emotions enter the conscious mind (balloon), it inflates even more and stress symptoms steadily worsen. These symptoms fall into four categories:

Physical symptoms: Pain somewhere in the body, such as headaches, chest pain, stomach pain, aches and pains all over the body, etc.; organ dysfunction, such as heart palpitation, difficulty breathing, nausea, diarrhea, etc.; and general body symptoms, such as exhaustion.

Emotional symptoms: Sadness, anxiety, panic attacks, etc.

Mental symptoms: Poor concentration, forgetfulness, confusion, slowed thinking, etc.

Behavioral symptoms: Irritability, angry outbursts, violence, acting out, abandoning family, etc.

If one asks this person, "How long have you had these symptoms?" he will say something like, "Oh, well, probably about three years, getting worse all the time." What this means is that his hidden mind reached its saturation point about three years earlier, and his balloon started re-inflating from then onwards. Unfortunately, most people do not seek psychiatric help until the balloon is about to pop ("I just can't take it any more!"), or until it has already popped ("I am very sick"). Now the patient becomes upset over his dreadful symptoms and sickness, and that adds more painful emotions into the balloon.

E. Low stress tolerance syndrome: As stress symptoms reappear one by one, the person is at a loss as to why he has them. He also notices that when he is upset about something, he stays upset. No matter what he does, he cannot calm himself down. Why? Because he can no longer bury emotions in his hidden mind and shrink his balloon. This person is known as *stressed-out*. His symptoms have been warning signals sent by his brain chemicals to his conscious mind, saying, *"Your soda bottle became saturated some time ago. Now your balloon is filling up with toxic, painful emotions. Get rid of them properly as soon as possible, damn it!"* However, the patient's focus now is on his increasingly uncomfortable stress symptoms, not his accumulating painful emotions. He puts these painful emotions out of his awareness. If you ask him, if he is angry, sad, hurt, etc., he would say, "Not at all!" He's like a person who has not noticed the gradual build-up of smoke in the house, and whose main focus is on how to switch off the screaming fire alarm. He would deny there is any smoke in the house.

Some of these symptoms, such as chest pain, are very frightening. The person thinks that a real physical disorder, such as heart disease, cancer, or stroke caused them. Stress is the last thing on his mind, since he has thought all along that he was coping well with whatever was upsetting him by being strong. To get quick relief from his dreadful symptoms, he abuses alcohol or drugs, which help to relieve his symptoms. Many of these people become alcoholics or drug addicts. If one goes to see a doctor at this point, the doctor might diagnose one as having a minor anxiety disorder or depressive disorder, and put him on a tranquilizer or antidepressant medication. This takes care of his symptoms and gives him some temporary relief. But the patient's problem is just beginning.

Over time, however, as more emotions accumulate in the conscious mind/balloon because of the inevitable stresses of daily life, the stress symptoms become worse. In addition, the painful emotions such as frustration and helplessness experienced in response to the unremitting symptoms themselves further inflate the balloon. *The severity of persistent symptoms depends upon the size of the balloon.* The bigger the balloon, the more stress symptoms there are. A person in this unfortunate predicament is said to be having *low stress tolerance syndrome* (see picture 14 below).

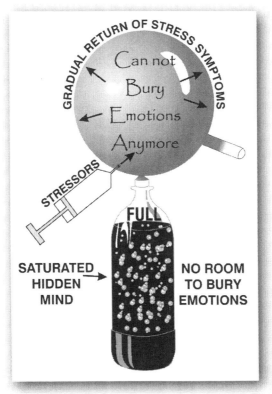

Picture # 14: Low stress tolerance syndrome: the balloon stays inflated.

Depending upon the size of one's balloon and the type of painful emotions in his balloon, the patient suffers from many stress symptoms: irritability, angry outbursts, sleeplessness, excessive sleeping, depression, anxiety, tension, poor concentration, inability to shut the brain down, a hundred different thoughts and emotions swirling in the mind, near-panic attacks, and many more. Depending upon the predominance of symptoms, people at this stage of stress are often diagnosed with minor stress disorders such as generalized anxiety disorder (GAD), Dysthymic disorder or chronic depression, Cyclothymic disorder (minor mood swings), attention deficit disorder (ADD), Fibromyalgia and the like. Their balloon could pop at any time. To prevent this from happening, these patients avoid all sensory stimulation, including people, commotion, traveling to distant places, watching television or anything that might upset them. They become increasingly withdrawn from social activities.

F. The breaking point: While all this had been going on, the brain chemicals have been changing in order to deal with the accumulating toxic, painful emotions in the brain. Finally, goaded by a *precipitating* or *triggering* bad event—the straw that breaks the proverbial camel's back—the emotional pressure in the conscious mind/balloon reaches its *breaking point*, and the balloon pops. The changes in the brain chemicals have finally resulted in a *chemical imbalance.* At this critical moment, the mind continually feels, "I just can't take it any more!" The stress symptoms have finally *crystallized* into a relatively well-defined stress disorder, such as major depression, panic disorder, etc. (see picture 15 below). Unable to tolerate emotional pain, many people in this predicament experience suicidal ideas.

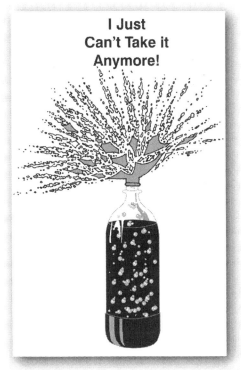

Picture# 15: The Breaking Point: a stress disorder is born.

G. The double whammy—a blast from the past: Some people's balloon pops suddenly and quite unexpectedly, and they are struck down with a major stress disorder like a bolt from the blue. In these people, a current painful event—say, the breakup of a relationship—brings into the conscious mind/balloon some painful emotions related to an old trauma buried deep in the hidden mind, such as being abandoned by one's mother or father in childhood. The fury of the painful emotions spewing from the hidden mind is so great that it pops the balloon (see picture 16 below). It is as if the soda bottle has been so vigorously shaken that fizz bursts into the balloon attached to the bottle's mouth. These people's soda bottles may not have been saturated at all, but they did hold, under pressure, painful memories of a very traumatic event in their past. Double whammy is a *blast from the past.* Sometimes, however, double whammy is milder in severity and causes only a few symptoms.

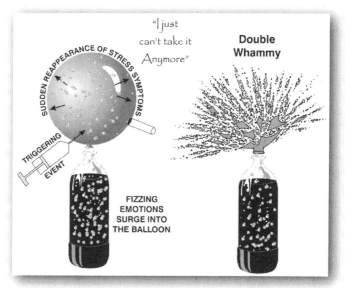

Picture# 16: The Double Whammy: buried emotions fizz up and pop the balloon.

H. Rule #2: The more severe the persistent stress symptoms, the less one is aware of the painful emotions in his mind and the stressors that caused them.

As the balloon begins to re-inflate and stress symptoms become worse, a curious thing begins to happen: the stressed-out person becomes more and more focused on his symptoms—sleeplessness, anxiety, poor concentration, panic attacks, depression, mind racing—and less and less aware of his inner, painful emotions and the stressors that caused them. People in this condition often make statements such as, "I don't know why I feel so miserable," "I don't know why I cry all the time," "I can't sleep a wink, and I don't know why," or "I have panic attacks, and nothing has happened to bring them on." If you ask the stressed-out person directly, "Is something bothering you?" he will answer, "Nothing at all, except my panic attacks!" If you ask, "What painful emotions are you having in your mind?" he will reply, "I have no painful emotions in my mind at all. The only pain I have is in my chest." If you ask, "Did something happen recently to upset you?" he will say, "I don't know what it could be. The only thing that happened to upset me was my headache attack!"

People whose balloons have popped and who are suffering from serious stress disorders, such as panic disorder or major depression, have almost no awareness at all about their blocked off emotional pain or the stressors that caused it. Their total focus is now on the symptoms of the stress disorder. This is no different from one's focusing on the screaming fire alarm, rather than on the smoke in the room.

How do we know that the stressed person's mind/balloon is full of painful emotions, and that he has been through many seriously bad events and problems? Well, as soon as the patient starts talking with a professional who is *sensitive, empathic, non-critical and non-judgmental,* he would break down and express his emotions—much to his own surprise. He would also reveal numerous horrendous events and problems that have traumatized him over the years. He would say, "I didn't know I had all these emotions in me and that I have been affected by all these bad events and problems." Raising one's awareness of the blocked off painful emotions in his conscious mind/balloon is the first and the most important step in learning to cope with stress. We studied in Chapter Three two cases of women who got well immediately after they expressed their highly painful emotions.

I. Medical Wild Goose Chase: Since some of these people do not know why they have their seemingly serious stress symptoms, they begin to run to doctors in a futile attempt to find an answer. They are now on a *medical wild goose chase,* in a perpetual state of bewilderment. We studied two cases of medical wild goose chase in Chapter Four.

Medical wild goose chase often has serious consequences. Some patients suffer from *medical trauma* as a result of mistreatment by the medical profession, and *fear of medications* due to reckless prescriptions given by inexperienced doctors and nurse practitioners.

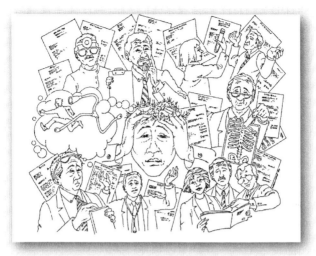

Picture# 17: Medical wild goose chase is demoralizing to patients and expensive for the national health care budget

Many of these patients suffer from three major emotional issues: dejection, disillusionment and demoralization. These hapless patients declare themselves as totally and permanently disabled, and apply for Social Security Disability. I must have evaluated over 5,000 of them for psychiatric evaluation between 1974 and 2010. They are a major drain on national health budget.

FIVE REASONS WHY PEOPLE BECOME STRESSED-OUT

The misery of stress and stress disorders, which millions of people in America suffer from, is preventable. It is based on the following five factors.

A. The lack of knowledge that the mind/brain/body is, in fact, one single unit, and painful emotions affect our body organs, and bring on frightening physical symptoms and serious disorders.

Ignorance of this single bit of information causes stressed-out people to ask such questions as, "How could my mind cause chest pain?" "How could stress cause my headache attacks?" "How could stress cause my heart to beat fast?" and to insist, "I am not imagining it! I am certain this is physical, not mental." They pursue repeated medical consultations with specialists to prove the point, and in the end, all they have to show for this *medical wild goose chase* is huge medical bills and three big Ds: dejection, disillusionment and demoralization.

What we think and how we feel affects every single organ in the body. Painful emotions in the brain can cause frightening physical symptoms without anything being physically wrong. Because of the intimate and intricate connections between the mind, brain and body, prolonged stress can bring on physical disorders, such as irritable bowel syndrome, arthritis, Fibromyalgia, high blood pressure, heart disease, chronic fatigue syndrome, psoriasis and many more. People who are unwilling to accept this reality are doomed to be on a medical merry-go-round for the rest of their lives.

B. The erroneous focus on physical activity as a solution for stress. Every single stressed-out person, regardless of his level of education, intelligence, profession or social status, belabors under the erroneous opinion that coping with and managing stress consist of doing something physical, such as jogging, exercising, taking hot tub baths or lifting weights. This focus on physical activities as a solution for stress symptoms is due to the fact that some of the most distressing stress symptoms are, indeed, physical, such as muscle tension and spasms, feelings of being "wound up," pain somewhere in the body, inability to relax, etc. However, this emphasis on *mindless* physical activity completely disregards the fact that stress is an emotional phenomenon. *Physical stress symptoms are caused by blocked off painful emotions in the mind.* Anyone interested in coping with stress must shift his focus from physical activity to learning to identify and deal with his blocked off painful emotions. This is extremely difficult for more stressed-out people. Here is an example:

> An intelligent white young woman with history of severe stress-related headache attacks attended one of my routine public seminars on stress. Throughout the 3-hour long seminar I repeatedly stressed that while physical exercise helped the body, unless one learned to deal with one's inner emotional pain, stress symptoms such as headache attacks won't go away. At the end of the seminar this woman approached and asked me, "Would jogging daily get rid of my headache attacks?" Obviously, she just could not accept the fact that she had to deal with her inner emotional pain for her to get rid of her headaches.

C. The use of inappropriate coping methods to calm down.
Almost all stressed-out people harbor the erroneous belief that

it is a *sign of weakness* to express their emotions, so they try to "be strong" when faced with stressful events and problems. When they are upset about something, they hide, bury or bottle up their painful emotions to calm themselves down. ("I don't want to think or talk about it. I just want to forget it!") When they can no longer hide their painful emotions, they indulge in denial ("I'm not upset. I have no problems."). They become experts in blocking their emotions off from their awareness. The unexpressed painful emotions get buried in the hidden mind and they disappear from their awareness.

Both these inappropriate ways of coping go utterly against nature. Their roots go back five thousand years, to when primitive man was being transformed into civilized man, and civilized society curbed the free expression of emotions as a way of taming primitive behavior. People who want to cope with stress must give up their hang-up about expressing emotions, and reject burying and denial as coping methods.

D. The habit of indulging in distractions to cope with pain promotes burying.

1. The most common distractions are *pleasurable* activities that millions of people indulge in: drinking alcohol to excess, abusing dangerous street drugs, smoking cigarettes, overeating, having promiscuous sex, gambling and overspending. These activities become bad habits that can lead to serious health, financial, family and legal problems. They block off painful emotions and promote the

burying of those painful emotions in the hidden mind. The hidden mind of just about every alcoholic and drug addict is saturated and his balloon is full.

2. When recreational activities, such as vacationing, hiking, trekking, skiing, cruising and the like are used to escape from having to deal with emotional pain, they also facilitate the burying process. These *avoidance* activities are, basically, an inappropriate response to stress.

A middle-aged white widow consulted me for chronic depression. History revealed that she lost her beloved husband in a car accident. Unable to deal with the stress of this tragedy, she went on a 6-week long cruise across the globe. This facilitated the burying process. Believing that she had coped with the tragedy by this distraction, she tried to move on with life. Gradually, her unfinished grief caught up with her and she became chronically unhappy.

E. The preference for the short-term benefit of drug treatment to the long-term benefit of learning better coping methods.
More and more people are resorting to *exclusive drug treatment* of their stress disorders due to the erroneous belief that their disorders are just the result of a chemical imbalance. They do not realize that unless they learn better coping methods, their stress disorders will keep getting worse over the years. Antidepressant drugs are also anti-stress drugs. However, they merely coat the surface of the mind/balloon and temporarily reduce the tension inside it; they don't shrink the balloon. *In fact, antidepressant drugs facilitate the burying process no different from alcohol and*

street drugs. In other words, these drugs give people a false sense of wellbeing and thus promote self-deception.

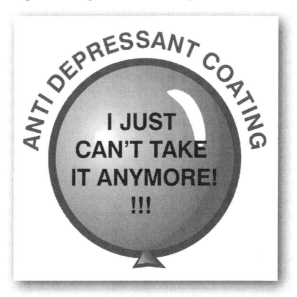

Picture# 18: Antidepressant drugs coat the balloon

As more emotions build up in the balloon, it pops again, and now one has a "breakthrough" episode of his stress disorder. He will then need two, three or even four drugs to coat the balloon and to control his stress symptoms. Most doctors prescribing antidepressant medication base their decision on a list of symptoms provided them by drug companies or DSM 5, rather than on adequate understanding of the stage of stress the patient is at, and the nature of stressful events and problems causing them.

Sometimes doctors add antipsychotic drugs to antidepressant drugs to 'augment' their effectiveness. All they are doing by this is to put a lid on the mouth of the soda bottle, and thus prevent the buried emotions from spewing up. (See picture 19 below).

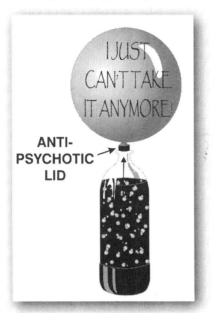

Picture# 19: Antipsychotics temporarily put a lid on the soda bottle

This strategy is good on a temporary basis. In the long run, however, they also stop working as life in full of bad events and problems, and these patients are unable to cope with them. This is how the 'refractory' and 'drug resistant' cases come into being.

Nowadays, doctors prescribe medications even to people who are merely grieving over the death of loved ones. In fact, the inappropriate and reckless use of antidepressant drugs by uninformed doctors is now so widespread that many patients are immune to drugs by the time they see a competent psychiatrist. Instead of learning to cope with stress, these patients are perpetually in search of new drugs to control their stress disorders. Drug companies are always eager to oblige them.

THE BEST TREATMENT MODALITY

Obviously the best treatment for stress and stress-related disorders is right combination of medication to alleviate symptoms immediately, counseling to release the pent-up painful emotions, and education for lasting benefit.

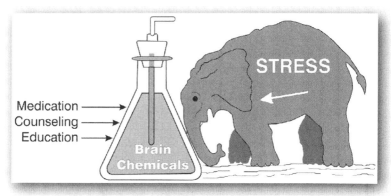

Picture#20: Judicious combination of drugs, counseling
and education works the best in the long run

SUMMARY: THE FIVE STAGES OF STRESS.

Now that the reader has a fair idea of what stress is here is a glimpse of the five stages of stress. At any given time, everyone in the world is in one of the following five stages of stress.

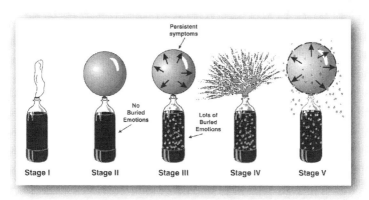

Picture#21: Five stages of stress

Stage One: Stage of Robust Health. The person in this stage is in good emotional and physical health. He has no maladies. He enjoys life to the fullest. He is a wise person who always *does the right thing.* He is a highly aware person. He is good at getting rid of painful emotions from his mind and solving his life-problems. He knows how to put things in proper perspective. He is adept at judging characters. He is able to change his perceptions. He uses humor to deal with difficult situations. He knows how to cancel-out or neutralize his painful emotions. He has good insight into his own mind. He lives a moral life. He has found *balance* in everything he does in life. His balloon is always shrunk. His soda bottle does not have many buried emotions. He does not abuse alcohol, drugs or indulge in other pleasurable things to cope with his everyday stress. Let me tell you, anymore it is harder and harder to find such people!

Stage Two: Stage of Distress. In this stage, an emotionally well-adjusted person is temporarily upset due to a particular event or problem. He is now called a *stressed* person. He has many stress symptoms. However, he is *fully aware* of why he is upset. If you ask him, he will readily tell you something like "I am upset because I lost my job," or "My mother died," or some such thing. He does not have any hang-ups about expressing emotions. His balloon is full of emotions, but his soda bottle does not have any painful emotions related to the current upsetting event. He can calm himself down relatively quickly by ridding his mind of painful emotions and solving the problem. If his current life situation is a little too overwhelming, he might benefit from one or two visits with a trained counselor. For example, a middle-aged man is unable to grieve over his mother's death because he has harbored some anger towards her. Once he talks out his anger, he grieves over the loss and goes back to being his normal self. *It is best to avoid medication treatment at this stage.*

Stage Three: Stage of Low Stress Tolerance. In this stage, the person is said to be stressed-out. His soda bottle is saturated, and he can no longer cope by burying his emotions. His balloon is inflated to varying degrees. He is unable to calm himself down. He is irritable, impatient, snappy and crabby. He is *not aware* of why he has these symptoms. His total focus is on his symptoms. If he sees a doctor, he will be diagnosed as having one or more minor stress disorders. At this stage, he may be helped by therapy alone in the hands of a very competent therapist if his stress symptoms are not too severe. However, most people seeking medical help at this stage end up taking one or more psychotropic medications. Most people at this stage respond well to medications. However, sooner or later they reach the breaking point and come down with a major stress disorder, unless they learn to shrink their balloon.

Stage Four: Stage of Stress Disorder. The balloon has finally reached its breaking point either due to gradual inflating of the balloon or double whammy. Because of a precipitating event, it has popped. Chemical changes in the brain have resulted in a *chemical imbalance,* and the diverse stress symptoms have crystallized into a relatively well-defined *stress disorder,* such as major depression or panic disorder. At this critical moment, the patient continually feels, "I just can't take it any more!" Psychodynamic counseling at this stage is generally useless, as the patient's suffering is so great that he has no awareness of his blocked off painful emotions. All he is looking for is quick relief from his numerous intolerable symptoms. Such patients need one or more drugs to control their symptoms. Even after they are treated with drugs, many of them just go back to the low stress tolerance stage (stage three). This explains why 30-50% of patients do not become completely symptom-free even with aggressive medication treatment. They must get counseling and education once they are fairly stable.

Stage Five: Stage of Despair. At this stage, the person has been through many successive breaking points resulting in *multiple* stress disorders: depression, panic disorder, psychotic disorder, high blood pressure, Fibromyalgia, irritable bowel syndrome, etc. The treatment process has probably traumatized him as well, and so he does not trust either therapists or doctors. He is fearful of drugs, or he is on multiple drugs for his multiple stress disorders. He has no clue, no trust, no hope and no desire even to try to get help. He has frequent suicidal thoughts. He considers himself totally and permanently disabled. He is constantly trying to get on some type of disability program. None of his healers seems to have a clue as to how he reached this stage of devastation.

The course of stress

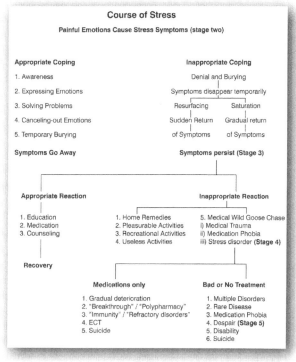

Picture#22

Part Two

My American Journey

New York Nightmare

OVER THE YEARS I HAVE come to the conclusion that one must endure American nightmare before achieving American dream. My nightmare began immediately after my plane landed in New York at 2.00 p.m. on June 26th 1970. I was a 25-year old fresh-from-medical-school doctor, impeccably dressed in a gray silk suit. That was the first time in my life I had worn a suit. On that day the sky was overcast and it rained intermittently. I took a taxi from JFK to Elmhurst General Hospital, paid $5 to the driver, picked-up my bag, and looked up to get a good look at the hospital I was to get my training over the next year. It was an imposing ten-story glazed pink brick building (Google image: Elmhurst Hospital Center).[12] I walked up the wet steps to the spacious lobby. A sign on the wall directed me to the Administrative Office to the left.

As I entered the office I saw several secretaries sitting behind their desks. None of them greeted me, none smiled. One of them

---

12   Today the building looks somewhat different. It now has two 'breasts' in the front.

asked me how she could help me. I told her that I had just arrived from India to join the hospital as an intern, and I needed a place to stay. She told me to wait, and left to get the hospital's Chief Administrator. After she returned to her table, she said, "He will be with you shortly." While waiting for the administrator, I tried to do some small talk. I showed her a photograph of my wife and myself and said, "We got married just three weeks ago!" She looked at it briefly and went back to work.

Soon a red-faced averagely built middle-aged white man with Abe Lincoln beard over his chin came towards me and shook hands with me. He said he was Mr. B. He did not smile. Nor did he welcome me.

Mr. B gave a quick look at my bag on the ground and asked me, "What can I do for you?" I told him I had just arrived from India and I needed a place to stay. He was not impressed.

"We have no place for you to stay here," he said curtly. "The residents' quarters are for residents on-call."

"The hospital brochure indicated that I could stay there for a few nights before finding my own accommodation," I said politely. "Sir, may I stay in the resident's quarters just for one night till I can find accommodation, please?"

"No," he said firmly. "The residents' quarters are only for residents on-call."

It was pointless to argue with this callous man. As I discovered four days later, what Mr. B told me was a blatant lie. Several new interns were already staying there. Till this incident, I had harbored the belief that Americans were compassionate, generous and helpful people. This crass behavior of a responsible hospital administrator was a rude awakening for me.

"How can I find a place to stay, Sir?" I asked him politely.

"You can look for an apartment around the hospital," he said curtly, and left. I did not know what all entailed in renting an apartment. Such was my ignorance having hailed from a small town in India. I learned later that to find an apartment, I needed to contact a real estate agency. I did not know what a real estate agency was. For, in India of those days, there were no real estate agencies. I found out soon that there was a real estate agency right in front of the hospital, but neither the sadistic Mr. B nor his indifferent secretaries volunteered that information.

By now it was 3 p.m. already. It was raining outside and I had no umbrella. I left my bag in the office and hurriedly went in search of an apartment in the neighborhood. I was already very hungry, and drenching in the rain made matters worse. Over the next one and one half hours, angry and hungry I went from one multi-storied apartment building after another near the hospital. They all displayed "no vacancy" signs. I knocked on several apartment units. People who opened doors for me seemed surprised to see me in my rain drenched gray suit asking, "Do you know any apartments for rent in this building?" Luckily none of them called the police on me.

By 4.30 p.m., I was totally frustrated and exhausted. I returned to the Administration Office and asked to speak to Mr. B again. He came out of his office looking somewhat irritated. Obviously, he could not care less that I had just arrived from across the globe and was hungry, cold, and drenched to my bones. I told him I had no luck finding an apartment. He told his secretary to give me the phone number of Y.M.C.A. and left in a huff.

He could have given me this information when we met earlier, but for some reason he had chosen not to.

I called the Flushing, N.Y., Y.M.C.A. and told the person on the line that I needed a room for a few nights. He said rudely, "We have no vacancy," and hung up. In less than 30 minutes the administrative office would be closed, and I would have to spend the night on the sidewalk. Desperate, I called Y.M.C.A. again.

"Sir, I have come all the way from India and have no place to stay for the night. Will you please give me a room even if it is just for one night?" He thought for a while and asked, "Do you have money?" I said, "Yes." He said, "Come on over."

"If this is the attitude of a 'Christian' Association, what can I expect from others?" I thought. I took a taxi to Flushing Y.M.C.A. and checked in. I gave the clerk three-day advance in cash. The man took me to a small room on the first floor. The room did not have an attached bathroom. I felt very relieved that at least I did not have to sleep on the sidewalk. I showered in the common bathroom, drank a glass of milk and went to bed.

To call Mr. B utterly callous and hateful is to pay him a huge compliment. Can you imagine an administrator of a hospital mistreating an intern who had just come all the way from India to serve his hospital?

However, my encounters with Mr. B. and Y.M.C.A. taught me two important lessons:

1. How I must *never* treat people who are in dire distress. This experience, happening on the very first day in a foreign land, when I was alone and utterly helpless, sensitized

me to the plight of lonely people in severe distress. A person without compassion for other people's suffering is unfit to be called human.

2. I realized that the Chief Executive Officer (CEO) of an institution sets the tone to the culture of that institution. My subsequent experience with employees of that hospital from top to bottom validated the age-old Indian adage: 'Like king like people.'

Many years later when I was the Medical Director of four psychiatric institutions, I made sure that all employees treated patients with compassion, respect and professionalism.

Over the years I met many compassionate and helpful Americans wherever I lived and realized that Mr. B was a sad symbol of how power could easily breed indifference and heartlessness in some people, and destroy their self-awareness and humanity. His cultivated evils must have masked whatever inherent godliness he might have in him.

When I woke up next morning, the sky was blue, sun was shining, the breeze was gentle and the world looked beautiful. I more or less recuperated from the previous day's ordeal. I ate a good breakfast and walked all the way to the hospital where I would be joining on July 1st. After familiarizing myself with the hospital's surrounding, I went to a nearby real estate office to look for an apartment. A young real estate agent helped me to locate a small studio apartment about ¾ mile from the hospital.

I went to the hospital on 30th of June to find out my assignment that would begin the next day. No one met with new interns to welcome or orient them to the hospital. The notice on the bulletin board revealed that my two-month long rotations through the hospital's various departments would begin with emergency department the very next day.

On the morning of July 1st, I went to the emergency room (E.R.). Dr. C., the Director of E.R., was a short, stern-faced, bespectacled, extremely hostile white man with curly hair. I never saw him smile even once. He did not want to know our names or where we came from. He was all business. He explained the rules and regulations of E.R. and said that he expected everyone to be there on time. He was more like a slave trader of 19th century than a doctor running the E.R. I thought that it was such a tragedy that this callous man without an iota of courtesy, good manners and compassion was a physician, and that, too, in the emergency room. I was relieved to notice, however, that he never put his hands on a patient. He simply sat in his small room and stared at us through a large glass window. Never once during my two-month stint in the emergency room did he come out of that room or teach anything to interns or residents. It was glaringly obvious that he was there just for his paycheck.

In the emergency room, Dr. C.'s assistant, a dowdy, middle-aged fat East European woman with strong accent "supervised" us. Her "supervision" consisted of going after interns and residents prodding them, "Quick! Quick! Move on to the next case. Move on!" Thank God, I never saw her even once touching a patient, or teaching anything to interns. Her role was that of a slave driver. The only thing her hands ever did was to constantly pull the edges of her undersized white coat to cover her bulging breasts. There was no teaching, no training, and no discussion of any patient. There was no time for such frivolous things, for at any given moment there were scores of patients in the waiting room.

Within two days it dawned on me that I was trapped in a slave labor camp. This city hospital needed warm bodies to fill the slots. Today this "training" would be considered as human trafficking. The hospital linked up with the famous Mount Sinai Hospital of New York only for the sake of attracting cheap labor on false premise. During the entire two months of service in the emergency room, I never once had the privilege of being taught anything by anyone –not even once. What little I learned was taught to me by the orderlies.

Treating overdose cases was completely new to me as this never happened in India. In India when people attempted suicide, they simply meant business. Either they hung themselves from the ceiling fan, or they drowned by jumping into the well or the river. Sometimes they drank rat poison. By the time they were brought to the hospital, they were all dead. The question of treating them in the emergency room did not arise. Truthfully, I had never heard of the term 'overdose.' I did not know how to put the lavage tube into the stomach to pump out drugs and wash it. An orderly taught me the trick. Soon I learned to stick the tube into the nose of the distraught patient and shout, "Swallow, swallow!" so that the tube would go into the stomach via the esophagus, and not into the lungs via the trachea. Again, a mater-of-fact orderly taught me how to lavage and remove toxic drugs from the stomach.

I was shocked by what I encountered in the emergency room. Gun shot wounds, stab wounds, head injuries, broken bones, mugging victims, overdoses, high fevers, heart attacks, strokes, meningitis... I was not prepared for most of these. Without proper support and guidance of superiors, I was completely at sea. I watched some Residents treat these cases, but they were too busy to teach us anything. I did what I could under the circumstances, thinking: "God help these poor patients!"

Thursdays afternoons were particularly dreadful as we saw dozens of middle aged ladies with broken heads, arms and wrists due to muggings by drug addicts. Thursday was the payday those days. Early hours of Monday mornings were also rather tense. We would wait in dread for numerous victims of heart attacks –people who dreaded going to work Monday morning! I thought to myself: "This is the legendary land of streets paved with gold where the whole world is dying to come! Over here people would rather die than go to work!"

Those were the days when Viet Nam war was raging. The whole nation was in constant turmoil. One could not turn the T. V. on without seeing gory details of dozens of American young men being killed in ambush, and hundreds of Viet Cong insurgent and innocent people being destroyed in bombing raids. "That is the way it is," said Walter Cronkite at the end of his tragic broadcast of CBS Evening News. Everywhere you looked you saw people in bellbottom jeans, wearing long beards and long hair in quiet protest against the war.

Many Viet Nam veterans who returned home became hippies, drug addicts and alcoholics. They often came to the emergency room to get narcotics. They showed up saying they had a small cut on the lip or hand. Obviously these wounds were self-inflicted, designed to get narcotics. They demanded morphine, codeine or Darvocet. If I refused, they would curse me up and down and swear to kill me when stepped out of the emergency room. Sometimes they made anonymous phone calls saying they had planted a bomb in the E. R. This required the E. R. to be evacuated promptly. This resulted in the overflow of the people waiting for service in the waiting room. Not a day passed without some horrible incident threatening the safety of the staff of the E. R. Disheveled hippies loitered the streets around the hospital aimlessly, symbols of the angry and disillusioned youth of America. The war in Viet Nam had come to America. Chickens had come back home to roost.

Initially the threats of these drug addicts to kill me frightened me quite a bit. I became rather paranoid every time I left the hospital. In fact, I called my wife before leaving the hospital saying, "If I am not home in fifteen minutes, call the police." However, after a while these threats got old. On one occasion, a burly, drunk black man in oversized colorful African-style shirt dragged his equally inebriated girlfriend to the E. R. and demanded that I perform a gynecological exam on her immediately. I was busy writing a note on the chart of a patient. Feeling ignored, the man slammed his massive hand heavily on the counter in front of me cursing me at the top of his voice. By now I had become somewhat immune to such threats. Without showing any emotion I clapped my hands and said loudly, "Guards! Guards!! Come here! Throw this rascal out!" At this, two big, uniformed

African American guards showed up, stood on either side of the offensive black man and said, "Let us go!" The man walked away cursing and threatening.

Then there were grownup children of elderly parents, who brought their parents to the emergency room with the avowed goal to have them hospitalized. The elderly parents on the wheel chair were in no physical or mental distress whatsoever. A few minutes of inquiry of the children revealed the true reason for their visit to the E. R. They were going on vacation abroad and their elderly parents needed someone to care for. Since Medicare paid for the hospitalization, the children would be spared the expense of babysitters.

When my wife came to New York in mid July, Dr. C. said refused me permission to go to the airport to receive her. I stood my ground. I explained to him that I had been married for only six weeks, and that my wife had never been abroad. Finally he grudgingly relented. I went to the airport and received my wife. Our marital life in America had just begun. Everyday during those early days I thought of returning to India. The problem was I had no money for the airfare. What a trap I had fallen into!

Following two months of posting in the Emergency room, I rotated in zombie-like daze through internal medicine, neurology pediatrics and surgery. I worked 36 hours straight and got only 12 hours to rest and recuperate. Most of the work I did was to draw blood around 5.30 in the morning, carry the vials to the laboratory, push patients to the X-ray rooms, start intravenous drips and do other menial tasks. I was in a daze most of the time with little time for meals, showers or sleep. On one occasion when I raised this issue with a hotshot internist, he said that they had all been through this themselves. He looked at me as though I was a whiner. To my relatives and friends back home, I was a big-time doctor in a "commanding position" at Mt. Sinai Hospital in New York!

Senior doctors were too busy checking blood tests and X-rays to even look at or talk with the patients. Everyone was in a great rush. Once in a while, an all-knowing attending doctor stood at the head of a patient's bed and the rest of us stood around it. Most of us were so sleepy that we listened with our eyes closed. The hapless patient lay there near death. No one said hello to the patient. Not a word of compassion passed from the lips of the internist to the ears of the patient. A resident presented the case as if the patient was deaf. The senior doctor would then ask about laboratory test results. He would then make some comments and move on to the next bed. If he chose to touch the patient's body for examination, he did not bother to ask the patient's permission. He simply put his hand on the patient's belly and poked around. By the time we were all through with the poking, most patients complained of soreness in their belly.

My medical training in India was mostly based on "detailed history, keen observation, gentle palpation, judicious percussion and careful auscultation." A doctor would have to depend on his intuition and experience to arrive at a diagnosis. To me being a doctor was being more an artist than a scientist. Blood tests, urinalysis, spinal tap and X-rays were ordered only to confirm the suspected diagnosis. In America the primary emphasis was on laboratory tests. I was shocked to note that I had to perform spinal tap on every single patient admitted with fever, no exceptions.

Besides being scientific, these tests were where the money was. In fact, most tests were ordered even before the doctor saw the patient. I simply could not make head or tail about all the test reports. Nor did I have time to read up on them.

During rotation through surgery, we were supposed to show up at 4 a. m. at the surgical theater. We would wash our hands with our eyes closed catching a little nap while washing hands. I have no idea what I did while assisting the surgeon operating on the patient. I wondered what the need was for operations to start 5 a. m. I wondered why couldn't operations start around 8 a. m.? Well, the sooner the surgeon was done with the surgery, the earlier he could go to his office and see more patients. It all boiled down to making money. The fast pace of life was driven by the need for money. There was no other reason for it.

During all this time, to my senior American residents I simply did not exist. Either they had nothing to say to me or they were totally oblivious to my presence in their company. For example, a senior resident began to flirt with a pretty nurse while I was just a step away from both. Neither of them behaved as if they were aware of the fact that I was a witness to their amorous exchanges. I was so insignificant in their mind that what I thought or felt mattered little to them.

The same was the case with another incident. A junior American resident punctured the rectum of an elderly man while performing colonoscopy on the ward. He panicked and left the ward abruptly leaving the hapless patient in bed. Soon the old man suffered from severe abdominal cramps, and came down with high fever due to peritonitis, inflammation of peritoneal lining of the intestines. This was a rather serious condition. The nursing staff called in a senior resident for an emergency consultation. When the senior resident was evaluating the patient, the junior resident showed up and jokingly said, "I kept pushing the scope up his rectum. Then suddenly I saw something bluish. Then I knew I had punctured his rectum." There was no remorse whatsoever in his tone for grievously injuring the patient and abandoning him. The senior resident just laughed with him. Neither of them seemed to be aware of the fact that I was right there watching the hideous drama right in front of the very sick patient. It simply did not matter what I saw or heard or thought for that matter. They all seemed to be oblivious to the fact that I was a human being just like them, even though different in color and appearance, with the same powers of the mind, the same powers of observation and judgment.

When I came to America I had thought that slavery ended over 100 years earlier. I realized that slavery was alive and well, though disguised as "medical training." The whole system was set up to exploit interns and residents and squeeze every last ounce of their blood. There was no humanity, no compassion, no kindness, no orientation, no training, nothing. This was my introduction to American medical system.

I will not trouble the reader with many other horror stories in this hospital except to say that it was like a war zone. I was not familiar with the American maladies brought on by excesses such as overeating. In India we treated mostly infectious diseases such as malaria, typhoid, cholera, etc. I could not learn about the

American maladies fast without anyone supervising my work and educating me.

Within 3 months of being in New York, I felt overwhelmed by situations both in the hospital and outside the hospital. Not a day passed without my regretting about having come to America. In October '70, I came to know that I had to start applying for residency position for the year 1971-72. However, I had no time to contact any other hospital. Those days there was no Internet, nor Google. Not knowing what to do, I applied for the position of first year resident of internal medicine at the same hospital, knowing well that I was utterly incompetent to occupy that position. I had learned absolutely nothing during the previous three months. Nor did I have time to read up journals. What little time I had outside the hospital, I spent recuperating and getting acquainted with compatriots in New York. The compelling reason for my applying for this post, however, was job security.

The hospital offered 13 first-year residency positions in Internal Medicine, and most positions usually went to Jewish or Christian interns of the U.S. and South America. Having ample support system in N.Y. City, they were quite at ease with the state of affairs. I knew that mine was a hopeless case. Nevertheless, Dr. Seckler, Director of Medical Education, gave me an appointment for an interview.

Dr. Seckler was a tall, thinly built, middle-aged bald Jewish man with a brownish French-cut beard. When I appeared for the interview at the designated time, he had just taken off his white coat and was putting on his plaid jacket. It was obvious that he was about to leave the office, perhaps before I showed up.

It became evident to me that the interview with me was merely perfunctory.

I apologized for interrupting his departure. He seemed embarrassed by his own behavior. He was honest.

"Well, the truth is that we have filled all the positions already."

"Well, that is all right, Dr. Seckler. No problem," I said. In fact, I was quite relieved that I did not have to work at the Elmhurst General Hospital the next year.

"Have you found a position elsewhere?" He asked me with a slight twinge of guilt.

"No. I am sure I will find one."

"Where all have you applied?"

"I haven't had time to apply anywhere so far. I have been too busy carrying blood samples to the laboratory, starting I.V.s and pushing patients to X-ray rooms." He must have sensed a tinge of sarcasm in my voice.

"Please sit down," he said taking off his jacket. "You don't like this hospital, I presume."

"No, I don't." I explained to him how disappointed I was with the "training program" in that hospital.

"If you are so disappointed with us, why did you apply for a position here?"

"Well, I had no choice. I had no time to apply elsewhere, as I have been too busy with 36-hour shifts. I must have a job to pay my bills, you see." No one ever talked with this man like this before. I had nothing to lose.

"Do you like New York?"

"No, I don't."

"Why? What is wrong with it?"

"Well, to a foreigner like me, New York seems totally heartless. It is a jungle out there. When I go to open a bank account, the officer asks me, 'What kind of account you want to open?' When I ask, 'What options do I have?' he appears frustrated. Everyone seems to be so stressed-out!"

"Why don't you like this hospital?"

I went on to describe to him all the stupid things I have experienced in the hospital from the day I entered the hospital lobby on June 26th, 1970.

"I have learned little since I joined this hospital. Most of my time is spent it drawing blood; taking the blood, urine and spinal tap fluids to the laboratories."

"You could summon the orderly to do all these things."

"Orderlies never show up in time. If I wait for them, the blood and spinal fluid samples would get spoiled, and I would have to do all these painful procedures again. So, I take them to the laboratory myself. The same is true with taking patients to the X-ray rooms. We simply cannot wait for orderlies to push gurneys to the X-ray department when the patient with head injury needs urgent X-rays. Besides, the elevators do not show up on time. So I have to carry the samples to the lab on the ground floor, and walk up six floors by the stairs. It is exhausting to do so dozens of times a day."

He listened to me intensely. And then he said, "Well, I am sorry you have found New York and this hospital so inhospitable. If there is any opening I will contact you."

"Please don't worry about me. I know I will find a position somewhere."

A week later I received a letter from Dr. Seckler offering me residency in Internal Medicine at Mount Sinai Hospital or City of New York. The letter read something like this:

Dear Dr. Kamath,

It gives me great pleasure to offer you the position of Resident in Internal Medicine for the year 1971-72 at the Mount Sinai Hospital Services, at City Hospital Center at Elmhurst, New York. I was quite impressed by our interesting discussion during your interview with me earlier this month. Congratulations!
David Seckler, M.D.

On the one hand, I was happy that I had the job for the next year. On the other hand, the letter scared the hell out of me, as I knew nothing about the job I was expected to do. Under the circumstances there was no way I could learn in the next 8 months whatever I was supposed to know to function as the first year resident in Internal Medicine. Then on January 2nd, 1971, an incident —actually an accident- happened that saved me from this predicament.

CHAPTER 9

The Accident

2 A.M. SATURDAY, JANUARY 2ND 1971. It had been exactly six months since I joined this hospital as an intern. I was fast asleep in the Resident's room in the hospital. The loud ringing of phone startled me from deep sleep, causing my heart to beat fast. For a moment I did not know where I was. I had just fallen asleep after working for 30 hours straight without a break. I was hoping to catch up with a few hours of sleep before the morning round of the wards beginning at 6 a.m. I did not know that the event that would happen in the next few minutes would change my life forever.

Before the second ring I reached out to the heavy black phone receiver, held it to my ear and, my eyes still closed under the weight of heavy eyelids, I whispered, "Hello." It was the nurse on the Internal Medicine ward. "Doctor Kamath, Mrs. Ross has pulled her I. V. out again. We had tied both her hands to the side railings as tightly as we could, and she still managed to pull it out! She certainly pulled a Houdini on us! You better come over and restart it." In this hospital, teaching interns to start intravenous drips was part of their "medical training." I just couldn't believe my ears. I had already restarted intravenous drip on Mrs. Ross several times before finally hitting the bed.

87-year old Mrs. Eleanor Ross suffered from a terminal case of lung cancer complicated by massive pneumonia. Cancer had ravaged her body to such an extent that now she hardly weighed 70 pounds. She had enjoyed a full life chain-smoking, drinking and running around. Now, she was just a lump of emaciated muscles, wrinkled skin and brittle bones. Her corrugated skin over both forearms bore large, dark purple-red blotches of blood due to numerous painful needle penetrations over the past two weeks. Starting I.V. didn't hurt her at all because much of her skin over her forearms and hands had died. But now she was tired of this whole game of early morning blood drawing and intravenous infusions. It was time for her to call it quits. So, every time I came to draw blood and start I.V. as ordered by my superiors, she begged me, "Doctor, please don't draw blood and start I.V. Please... let me die in peace. Please... I beg you."

During the years of my medical education India in late sixties, a terminally ill patient such as Mrs. Ross did not have to beg to be allowed to die peacefully. It was everyone's birthright to die in peace. The philosophy that guided this dignified approach to dying was based on 4000-year old 'The Great Death-conquering Mantra'[13]: *O three-eyed Lord, just as a gardener severs ripe melon*

---

13 Rig Veda: Mahā Mrithyunjaya Mantra: 7:59:12. This is one of the most sacred Mantras (magical hymns) from Hinduism's earliest sacred book Rig Veda (1500-1000 B.C.). The three-eyed Lord in this hymn is said to be Shiva, one of the three great deities of Hinduism. In the Triad of Great Gods of Hinduism, he is the God of destruction.

from its bondage to the vine, liberate me from (the cycle of birth and) death and grant me immortality.

The philosophy that guided this passive approach to death was, "Let the ripe fruit fall!" People get old, they become ill, and they die. This is the Law of Nature. There is time to be born, time to enjoy life and time to say goodbye. In India of my medical school days, terminally ill patients such as Mrs. Ross did not receive any heroic treatment. Being a part of the *death-accepting culture,* doctors allowed them to die with dignity. There was a time when, realizing that their time had come to depart this world, old people simply went to some holy place to die so they won't be a burden on their poor families.

But now I was in America, and doctors over here were part of a *death-defying culture.* Americans allegedly valued life more than the Easterners did. However, if one watched the Western movies, for that matter any American movie, one would come to the opposite conclusion. The heroes killed people like they were flies.

During one of our rounds, I said to my senior white American Resident, "Mrs. Ross has lived a full life. She just wants to die in peace. Why can't we just let her go?" The pompous resident looked at me in askance and said, "This is America. Over here we value life. We have a moral responsibility to keep Mrs. Ross alive no matter what." That was that. I could say no more about this. It did not bother him that we were torturing Mrs. Ross inhumanely in order to keep her alive. This reminded me of the policy the American army followed during the Viet Nam war: *Let us burn down the villages of poor people to save them from the Viet Cong!*

However, the ideal of sanctity of life had a darker side. Mrs. Ross was an important source of revenue to this sanctimonious hospital. Aside from billing Medicare for her daily care, the hospital billed Medicare for laboratory tests, X-rays, I.V.s, spinal taps, medicines, and every little act in saving her from death. The longer she was kept alive the more Medicare money the hospital stood to make. This was the proverbial elephant in the room.[14] Besides all this, Mrs. Ross was a guinea pig for interns and residents to receive their "medical training." No wonder Mrs. Ross preferred death to this torturous "treatment." The concept of hospice was still several decades ahead.

Now, at 2 a.m., it was my task to destroy Mrs. Ross's desire to die and snatch her away from the jaws of death. I dragged myself out of the bed, went to the main building, took the elevator to the sixth floor, and went straight to the broad corridor leading to Mrs. Ross's ward. The ward held five beds on either side, each separated by series of screens. Approaching Mrs. Ross's bed I said in irritation, "You did it again, Mrs. Ross, didn't you?" She half-opened her eyes and said in a faltering voice, "Doctor, please… let… me… die… in… peace. I beg you, please don't start I. V. I just don't want to live anymore. Please!" Ignoring her pleas I looked closely at both her hands and forearms. They were almost completely blue due to spilling of blood under her skin. She had been stuck so many needles over the past two weeks that now her veins were all clogged up with clotted blood. All I could feel were thin hard cords along her emaciated forearms.

---

14 It took Medicare officials another fifteen years to catch up with this scam and come up with the system of DRG –Diagnostic-related Group. According to this plan Medicare paid a fixed fee for the treatment of a given diagnosis regardless how many blood tests and X-rays were ordered. Suddenly the number of tests doctors ordered decreased.

I looked at Mrs. Ross and said to her, "Mrs. Ross, I wish I did not have to restart your I.V. But I have to follow orders of my senior doctor. I have been told by my resident to keep you alive no matter what. I have no choice but to restart your I.V. Please cooperate with me."

"I had to follow orders of my superiors!" Haven't we heard that excuse from Nazi soldiers following World War II?

Mrs. Ross shook her head in protest. She pulled both her restrained wrists with the greatest strength her frail body could muster and tried to wriggle her wrists out of the knots of gauze restraints around them. She pleaded, "Let me go. Please! Let... me...go!"

The nurse and I pulled her left forearm back to the bed and tied it securely again to the side railing. Mrs. Ross tried to fight us with her right arm. We tied her right wrist securely to the handrail on the right side by a thick gauze belt. I then inserted the needle into her left forearm groping for a vein that might still be open. All the while the feisty Mrs. Ross kept fighting us with the last ounce of energy in her frail limbs. Finally, after five minutes of groping the needle under her dead skin, I got the I.V. restarted. I taped the needle securely to her forearm and let the fluid run into her vein. "Thank God!" I said, "Mrs. Ross, now you can relax and go back to sleep."

At this, Mrs. Ross, let out a loud scream as if she was determined to fight me till her last breath. She arched her whole body pushing her belly as far up in the air as possible, turned her body to the left and pulled her right arm with such strength that the restraint of her right arm somehow loosened and before we could catch it she grabbed the I.V. tube with her right hand. She pulled on the I.V. so strongly that the needle, which had been firmly taped to the dying skin with tapes, began to come out of the vein. I grabbed her right hand, held it firmly in place so the needle would not come out. I said angrily, "Stop it, Mrs. Ross! Stop it! Let it go! Let it go, Mrs. Ross!"

This time around Mrs. Ross was determined to fight me to the end. She kept pulling the I.V. I was desperate. I did not know what else to do to prevent the I.V from coming out. Instinctively I pinched hard the skin over the back of her right hand and squeezed it as hard as I could, hoping that the pain would make her let go. All the while I found myself shouting, "Stop it! Stop it! Mrs. Ross! Stop it!" I had forgotten that Mrs. Ross was beyond experiencing pain. The skin over the back of her right hand had died long time ago.

Suddenly I found myself holding a large chunk of Mrs. Ross's dead skin between my forefinger and thumb, revealing the red, raw inner layer of skin over the back of her right hand. I was taken aback by this surreal event. I kept looking at the chunk of dead skin in my hand. For a moment I was in a daze. I looked at the nurse as if seeking her sympathy with my inhumanity. I noticed neither horror nor disapproval on her impassive face. Perhaps she had become callous to such dehumanizing horrors in her daily routine. For once I became aware of how I had lost my humanity within six months of beginning my "medical training." Now I had become the bona fide member of the callous New York City Hospital System. The "medical training" I was getting had little to do with healing people. This whole farce was strictly a business. It had everything to do with making me the callous doctor who could look at patients impassively, unmoved by their immediate suffering. There were larger issues at play than the mere suffering of a little old lady with terminal cancer. Now I knew the real meaning of the axiom: *America's business is business!*

I gently placed the dead skin over the raw area and put a gauze bandage over it. I turned the I.V. flow off and pulled the I. V. out of the vein. I cut loose all the restraints. Bringing my face very close to Mrs. Ross's left ear, I put my hand gently over her forehead and said to her, "Mrs. Ross, today it is my privilege to grant you your wish to die in peace. I will not torment you any more."

Mrs. Ross looked at me with gratitude in her eyes. She whispered, "Thank you, doctor! Thank you!" I looked at the nurse meaningfully and said to her, "I don't want to torture her any more. Pull this screen around Mrs. Ross. Call me when she has passed away." The nurse nodded understandingly. I left the ward with a heavy heart and went to bed around 3 a.m.

My phone rang around six a.m. It was the end of the night shift for the nurse. The nurse said, "Dr. Kamath, Mrs. Ross died peacefully five minutes ago. You need to stop by and sign the death certificate." I went back to the medical floor and checked on Mrs. Ross. She was dead. The night nurse had the death certificate ready for me to sign. We exchanged meaningful glances for a fleeting moment. I signed the death certificate and walked to my studio apartment in a daze.

I went to bed around 8 a.m. Though very tired, I could not fall asleep. The events of the early morning hours haunted me.

This was not an isolated incident that had shocked me during this period of "training." This was but just the tip of the iceberg, the epitome of what, in my mind, was wrong with American medical system. This "medical training" had bred callousness to human suffering in me. This was not the medical training I had expected when I came to America from India six months earlier. Now I knew the true meaning of the phrase "challenging position" in the hospital's advertisement offering internship positions in the Directory of American Hospitals. This phrase stood for, for lack of a better term, slave labor. It was clear to me that this hospital was ill equipped to train foreign medical graduates (FMG).

Now, after the horrendous incident with Mrs. Ross I had second thought about continuing to work at this hospital in the coming years. The incident with Mrs. Ross was the straw that finally broke the proverbial camel's back. I concluded that the "medical training" I was getting at the E.G.H. not only did nothing to make me a better doctor, but also did everything to make me a bad human being. I simply had to get away from this horrible situation and madness of New York City.

The incident with Mrs. Ross crystallized in my mind that a career in Internal Medicine, at least as I knew it then, was not my cup of tea. One must be a masochist to pursue this path, I thought.

After two fitful nights of sleep in my own bed that weekend, I went to Dr. Seckler's office. I gave back to him the appointment letter I had received from him about a month earlier and said, "I do not wish to join your residency program for Internal Medicine for the year 71-72. Please give this position to someone else."

Dr. Seckler became very angry with me. He said, "Well, young man. I think you need some psychiatric help. I think you should see my psychiatrist friend Dr. W. whose office is on the first floor."

"Yes," I said. "I better see a psychiatrist before I become completely insane!" I left his office feeling insulted. But he was right. I had reached my breaking point.

Indeed, the ordeal of internship and life in New York had taken a toll on my mental as well as physical health. I suffered from bouts of stiff neck and pain in the pit of my stomach. I could not go to shopping centers without feeling anxious and severe pain in the pit of my stomach. Whenever I entered a shop, the sales person followed me around as if I would steal something. I could not blame him for this, as shoplifting was common and colored people were not trusted. However, it offended me a great deal as I considered myself as honest beyond reproach. The salespeople suspected me even more when he saw me pressing my stomach with my hand to alleviate pain. When going home after work, I had to constantly look over my shoulders for fear of being mugged. I suffered from other stress symptoms also such as irritability, fitful sleeping and overeating. My suffering from these stress symptoms sensitized me to the suffering of my psychiatric patients in the years to come. At the same time, I was aware of the connection between these symptoms and the real problems causing them.

The silver lining in the gloomy sky of New York life was that we met two couples in New York, who were from our hometown in India. They were like elder siblings for us. Balu Pai and his wife

Vijaya as well as Dr. Mohan Shenoy and his wife Lalitha made us feel at home by their wonderful hospitality. Shenoys even gave us Diwali oil bath in November! They made our New York nightmare more tolerable.

Regardless, as advised by Dr. Seckler, I went to Dr. W.'s office near the emergency room. He was a small, bespectacled man in white coat. He was so busy that he did not even ask me to come into his office. He stood across the high counter at the reception and asked me why I was there. I told him, "I gave up my position as resident for the coming year. I just didn't like the training program here. Dr. Seckler thought I had some psychiatric problem. He told me to see you." I explained to him that I just could not reconcile myself to the kind of medical training I was getting at the hospital, and I had to get away from here. At this he made an empathic statement: "I understand. If you don't like it, just switch to some other specialty. Just don't worry about it. Move on." I felt better right away. My brief contact with this psychiatrist made me realize the power of understanding and empathy, and it helped me to regain my sense of balance. I decided I would take up psychiatry as my specialty. I thought this specialty suited my temperament and met my need to have some *emotional connection* with the people I was to heal. So the first "emotionally troubled" person I ever met was myself. This experience gave me the ability to empathize with people who suffered from one psychiatric disorder or another, and through personal suffering I came to know what stress was.

Granting Mrs. Ross her wish to die and giving up residency position were two feeble acts of defiance on my part when I faced a powerful adversary. Had I continued to be part of that culture, my dilemma would have been over, but then I would have become very much like the many doctors I met over the years in connection with my little son's leg surgeries –cold, indifferent and utterly oblivious to the child's or parents' suffering.

Victor Frankl, a neurologist, psychiatrist, holocaust survivor and author, said: *The way in which a man accepts his fate and all the suffering it entails, the way in which he takes up his cross, gives him ample opportunity – even under the most difficult circumstances to add a deeper meaning to his life.*

CHAPTER 10
Jumping from the Fire Into the Frying Pan

You might think that I wrote the above cliché in reverse. No. That was what really happened. I was destined to sizzle on a frying pan for the next three years before I was done medium well.

Once I made the decision to pursue psychiatry as my vocation, I began feverishly to apply for training programs at various nearby psychiatric hospitals. The first hospital to offer me an interview was Hillside Hospital in Queens, New York. The interview went well. I was offered a position. However, when I asked if I could rent one of their on-site apartments meant for the Residents, the Director said that they had already been allocated. Even though the Hillside psychiatric training program was highly rated, I decided not to accept the offer, as I simply could not think of learning anything when I had no decent place to live, and I had no car to drive around. Clearly, I was operating on *survival mode.*

Next I applied at the New York State Psychiatric Hospital at Yonkers, N. Y. Again, I had the same experience: "Yes, we can offer you a position, but we have no place for you to live on the premise. They have all bee allocated." Then I applied at Connecticut Valley Hospital at Middletown, Connecticut. This time I was in luck. I took the Greyhound bus to Middletown, CT. for an interview. The program director, who came to receive me at the Greyhound bus station, was a congenial elderly balding gentleman by the name of Dr. Prins. He was born and raised in Holland, he said in his thinly disguised European accent. He had joined the hospital many years earlier and was now a fixture at the Hospital. He not only offered me a position with the residency training program, but also a small cottage on the sprawling hospital campus. What I did not know was that all State Hospitals were merely warehouses for chronically ill schizophrenics, and they hardly offered any training in psychiatry. Like Elmhurst General Hospital, the "training program" in this hospital was also designed to attract warm bodies for slave labor. All senior staff members were those who had graduated from State Hospital psychiatric training programs and they did not know a damn thing about psychiatry other than drugging up very sick schizophrenics.

Connecticut Valley Hospital was one of the oldest psychiatric State Hospitals in the country. The hospital consisted of numerous old buildings, some over one hundred years old, which stood on a tree-studded 100-acre campus overlooking the Connecticut River. The sprawling green lawn was dotted with tall, leafy trees, and we could see all around in the distance little hills and dales. Many years ago, the hospital housed over five thousand patients. These patients were all products of Industrial Revolution. The hospital campus was like a small city by itself. In fact the campus even had a police station and post office on the premise. As Dr. Prins drove me around the campus, he explained that over the past few years the number of inpatients had steadily gone down mainly due to improved drug therapy of serious psychiatric disorders, and better outpatient resources. As we drove by some of the buildings, I could hear screams of psychiatric patients emitting from them. The thought crossed my mind, "Is this what I can look forward to come July?" However, this place of screaming patients seemed far better than the mind-numbing madness of E.G.H. as well as New York City. Solely on the basis of getting a place to live near the work place, I chose to move to Middletown, CT. I signed the contract for the three-year psychiatric training program. I returned to New York City to complete my internship.

I finished my internship in Elmhurst General Hospital on 30th June 1971. I had no transportation to Middletown. I thought of renting a car, but I was really scared to drive on expressway even though I had the license to drive. I had never driven a car except the student-training car. Dr. Mohan Shenoy insisted that I should not drive, and he dropped us off at Middletown, CT. I credit him with saving my life. We became lifelong friends. I joined the training program on July 1st 1971.

CVH was built in 1868 and was originally named Connecticut General Hospital for the Insane. It was one of the first psychiatric facilities in the U. S. In fact, there were still decrepit old buildings on the premise, which had iron rings and chains riveted into the walls –evidence of inhumane treatment many patients received there consistent with the then mode of treatment known as Moral

Treatment. Now all patients were confined to relatively modern buildings.

In the early part of 20ᵗʰ century, the hospital became famous when a former patient named Clifford Whittingham Beers wrote the book titled, 'A Mind That Found Itself: An Autobiography,' published in 1907. A Yale graduate, Mr. Beers was committed to Connecticut State Hospital for the Insane for one and a half years after suffering from a manic episode. Much of his book described the atrocities he witnessed at the hospital - poor conditions, abusive staff, and lack of therapy. After its publication, his book stimulated a nation-wide movement to reform the State Hospital treatment of patients. The book revolutionized institutional care by making it the *last* resort, instead of the first resort as advocated by the theory of "moral treatment." Beers went on to found the Connecticut Society for Mental Hygiene, which helped prevent people from entering institutions, as well as providing after-care for discharged patients.[15]

I settled down in a comfortable two-bedroom house on the hospital premise, not far from the building where hundreds of screaming chronic schizophrenics were warehoused. In fact, visitors to my house were taken aback by the screaming they heard. When I visited the ward, I realized that this was nothing but a bedlam. Dozens of seriously ill patients ran around, sometimes half or fully naked. There was a certain smell that emanated

---

15   Exactly one hundred years after Mr. Beers published his book, Department of Justice investigated CVH, and in its report dated August 6, 2007 cited it for numerous civil rights violations and inadequacies in patient-care. Goes to show that it is almost impossible to reform State Hospital System due to poorly trained entrenched staff.

throughout the building, clearly one of body fluids mixed with disinfectants used to clean the floors. It was obvious that these patients did not get proper drug treatment to control their bizarre behavior. Clearly, this was a cuckoo's nest.

The superintendent of the hospital, Dr. A was a congenial immigrant psychiatrist in his mid forties. He was most gracious to all the new residents, and what a contrast it was from the reception I received in New York a year earlier! He invited all new recruits to his beautiful house on the hospital premise and threw a welcome party. He served us a lot of wine. I was not used to drinking alcohol, and so when I left his house, I was quite drunk. I drove recklessly to my cottage in a state of severe inebriation. Luckily, I was not arrested. I was totally ignorant of the consequences of drunk driving. I was penniless myself, and so I borrowed $50 from Dr. A., which I returned to him after I received my first paycheck. Looking back, it was such a stupid thing to do, but he being an Easterner like me, he knew that I did not know my boundaries.

In those days, ignorance of psychiatric disorders was such that just about everyone admitted to the hospital was diagnosed with schizophrenia. The only treatment was to drug them all up with one to three antipsychotic drugs. Psychiatric diagnoses were simply divided into psychosis and neurosis. We were told that the difference between the two was that whereas neurotics distorted reality, psychotics were out of touch with it. Regardless, the treatment was the same. Just drug them up. I could not make out the difference between the two.

There was a well-entrenched system in place that was basically run by a few nurses and orderlies. The situation was not much different from 64 years earlier when Mr. Beers published his book. These nurses and orderlies knew what medications helped patients the best. For example, a nurse would call me and say, "So and so is acting up. We have her in a straightjacket. I would like to give her a shot of Nembutal." It was more of an order than request. Most likely, the shot had already been given. The staff put patients in a straight jacket whenever they wished. They were very good at keeping law and order on the ward. They were used to seeing ignorant psychiatric Residents like me come and go. Any patient who resisted would pay for his impertinence sooner or later: Straightjacket and shots of Nembutal. Some patients seemed to enjoy these "comforts" offered by the "concerned" staff. It was all for their own good, you see.

A few psychiatrists were assigned to "supervise" our training, but it did not take long for new residents to figure out that they knew next to nothing about psychiatry. However, they knew how to prescribe drugs to patients. A privately practicing American doctor by the name of Dr. Robins was an old fixture in the hospital. He came everyday, saw some patients, prescribed them drugs and left after an hour or so. He was the one who told me about the difference between neurosis and psychosis. An Irish doctor by the name of Dr. Byrne came everyday, held a staff meeting in which all the new patients were interviewed –interrogated would be a better term. Dr. Byrne was a good-humored man in his mid forties. He basically did what he was supposed to do. All his notes were the same: *The patient's affect is flat and inappropriate; the patient displayed looseness of association and thought blocking; the patient displayed bizarre delusions and auditory hallucinations.*

Whether the patient actually had these symptoms or not mattered little, as the treatment was the same anyway: Just drug them up. It was clear that Dr. Byrne had no clue as to what the heck he was doing. He did hold an impressive smoking pipe in his hand, which he stuck between his lips from time to time. Day after day, I sat through this ritual. All other staff members did their part dutifully. The social worker, one wonderful, prim and proper elderly lady by the name of Babcock, diligently took notes and met with the family regarding placement of patients following their discharge, and the like.

Dr. Byrne had a large family that lived not too far from my house. One fine morning he packed his bags and left for Ireland. Perhaps he went back home to write a book titled, 'A Mind That Lost Itself.' Once in a while a "teaching staff" member held a lecture of some sort, which made little sense. One could make out that psychiatry was a great mystery to him also.

Once in a while we were graciously allowed to attend a lecture by a great local psychiatrist. There was one charismatic doctor by the name of Dr. Gladstone. He had some definite ideas why people became schizophrenic. He blamed it all on the parents. He interviewed parents of schizophrenics in front of students. He would ask them how they divided their responsibilities at home. When the father said, "I take care of major things and my wife takes care of minor things," he made a joke about it as if that was a terrible thing to do. He said that this "confusion" was what caused their child to become schizophrenic. The crowd responded to his joke and gave out a big laughter much to the embarrassment of the hapless parents. I knew nothing about schizophrenia or mental illnesses, but commonsense told me that there must be more to schizophrenia than just this. Looking back, all these great guys I came into contact with were groping in darkness themselves. The blind led the blind in pitch darkness.

I was on-call once every three nights. When state troopers or Sheriff's Deputies brought a legally committed patient to the hospital, I interviewed him or her. Again, I blindly followed Dr. Byrne's formula. However, I was kind to the patients. I asked them simple questions not knowing what to look for. I did not have anyone supervising my work. So, I just gave the patients drugs other doctors gave to their patients. Most patients got better, their psychotic symptoms such as delusions and hallucinations abated, and they went home on drugs. What happened to them after their discharge was anyone's guess. Many of them returned after a few days or weeks. This cycle of admission and discharge, known as the 'revolving door,' was standard with all State Hospitals. I was amazed, however, by the fact that so many severely psychotic patients improved within a few days, and seemed almost normal. I deluded myself that I was a good doctor.

The psychiatric residents' exposure was mostly to these "terminally ill" psychotic inpatients. Once in a while we went to an Outpatient Clinic in a nearby town and saw people with "neurotic" disorders, such as patients suffering from depressive and anxiety disorders, but we had no idea what these disorders were. We did not get any didactic instruction about mental health and mental disorders. Our daily routine consisted of going to the wards, assessing patients for psychotic symptoms, adjusting their medications, and then goofing off. I knew that with this type of training, I would not be able to practice psychiatry once I completed it.

Then the Director of Training Dr. Prins retired. One of the supervising psychiatrists was appointed in his place. This gentleman was himself in darkness about psychiatry as he once confessed to me in private. He had received his training in a State Hospital such as this. Occasionally he gave a lecture on some topic, which made no sense to most of us, and to him as well. I realized that I knew less psychiatry than the orderly on the floor. In fact, I often relied on their judgment as to what drug to give the patient. Sometimes when I checked the chart, I found out that a senior doctor who worked on the floor had changed the medication without discussing with me, or teaching me why he did so. When I tried to learn from him, he confessed to me that he knew only two drugs well. So whenever I gave patients any other drug than those, he changed the drugs to those that he was familiar with.

One year passed like this. I had my fill of mental rest. It dawned on me that I had jumped from the fire into the frying pan. I had learned absolutely nothing about my chosen field. The real problem was that there was not much to learn as modern psychiatry was still in its infancy. Freud's psychoanalytic theories were totally irrelevant in the treatment of psychotic patients in the hospital setting. In fact, they were useless in modern America even for the treatment of 'neurotic' patients except for the concept of 'the unconscious mind.' This was what I later called the 'hidden mind,' the soda bottle with the dissolved fizz. Drug treatment was in its early stages, and still evolving. There were hardly half a dozen psychotropic drugs in the market. I wondered what my own future would be if this was going to be my "training" for the next two years. I would be woefully unprepared to take up any responsible job outside the State Hospital milieu. I would be the proverbial frog in the dry well.

One angry American resident's complaints about the woeful quality of the training program fell on deaf ears. Increasingly he came across like an Aflac duck. When he escalated his protests, the administration summarily dismissed him from the program. Shocked, he came to the rest of us and pleaded with us to support him in his effort to reform the training program. We were all confused and scared to do anything as we were afraid of being dismissed as well. Being a foreigner in America, I felt highly vulnerable to dismissal and deportation if I created too much trouble. In September 1972, I applied for 3rd year resident's position at a private hospital nearby. The interviewer was so shocked by my ignorance that he was speechless. He dismissed me politely, and I drove back home in tears.

Around October 1972, the Joint Commission of Accreditation of Hospital (JCAH) came to inspect the hospital. In the course of their inspection, they interviewed two residents-in-training for feedback on the training program. The first one was Dr. M., a female American resident. Fatefully, the second one the hospital administration chose to meet with the JCAH team was myself. Perhaps Dr. A. mistook my fearful passivity to complacency. Apparently Dr. M. told the inspectors that the training she received satisfied her. When my turn came, I expressed serious concerns about my future. I explained that I had learned nothing so far in the hospital training program. I had not the slightest idea what I was doing there.

Baffled by the discrepancy between what I said and what Dr. M. said, the JCAH team re-interviewed Dr. M. Once she knew that the cat was out of the bag, she recanted her story and confessed that the whole program was a sham. Immediately the JCAH withdrew its certification and threw the whole hospital in chaos. The superintendent was furious. He met with us all in a small room. Looking at me straight, he kept saying, "You are in denial." My ignorance of psychiatry was so profound that I did not know what the term 'denial' meant. I just sat there and listened to his rant impassively. He taught me the lesson that when the top man is well entrenched in a rotten system, he becomes complacent as well as oblivious to the fact that he is swimming in a cesspool.

Luckily, the JCAH ordered the hospital to become affiliated with Yale University at New Haven, just thirty miles to the west. In January 1973 we were sent to train at the Community Mental Health Center (CMHC) in New Haven. This was the first CMHC established in the United States. We were assigned a supervisor by the name of Dr. Laub. He was a wonderful teacher, though in an abstract way. I interviewed patients and later discussed the interviews with him. Even though Dr. Laub did not give us any didactic lessons, discussion of patients and the symbolic ways by which they expressed their inner pain helped me to get a glimpse of psychiatry. Another gentleman was Dr. Geller, a psychologist who was very perceptive. The eighteen months I spent at CMHC was the turning point in my life. For the first time in two and one half years in America, I thought I finally met people who knew what they were talking about. I also had occasion to listen to the lectures of great psychiatrists of the time such as Dr. Theodore Lidz and Dr. Steven Fleck. What both of them said was way beyond my grasp, but being in their presence itself was uplifting. Dr. Balsam, Dr. Garber, Dr. Flamm, Dr. Glasser, the neurologist, and many others supervised me. Once in a while I met with a private psychiatrist by the name of Dr. Zentner in Hartford, CT. Even though most of what I heard from them was well beyond my comprehension, I absorbed what little I could like a dry sponge. However, none of them spelled out how the mind worked. Each patient was a distinct entity, and getting to know each one was like reinventing the wheel. Looking back, I must have come across to my supervisors as a total idiot. Had I been in their position, I would have taught psychiatry to residents in a more concrete way like I did to my private patients years later –on a white or black board. Nothing imparts knowledge to students better than private audiovisual presentation of a case under study. During my private practice, using the model of the mind I could teach my patients in one session more psychiatry than what all these supervisors taught me in scores of supervisory sessions.

During this time two incidents happened that gave me some insight into my own mind. On October 3rd 1973, when I went to CMHC as usual, I was told that Dr. Laub had left for Israel to fight Yom Kippur War. I had heard that morning that a terrible war had broken out in the Middle East and a lot of people had died. For once I feared for Dr. Laub's safety. I had come to like him very much, for he was so kind and empathic. Suddenly, however, I found myself feeling very calm. Next thing I knew, I felt as though I was a brilliant psychiatrist myself like Dr. Laub. When I met with my colleagues, I talked to them as if I was him and they were my students. I analyzed just about anyone I came across. My bossy behavior was quite out of character, and my colleagues detested me for it. For three days I was insufferable, a plain horse's arse. I was irritable and critical of others. Obviously, unbeknownst to me, my balloon had fully inflated due to anticipatory grief. On the fourth day, while I was on my way home from New Haven, suddenly I felt like crying. I let out my emotions and wept all the way to Middletown, thinking of Dr. Laub. Immediately I felt better. After Dr. Laub returned to work safe and sound, I shared this experience with him. This personal experience of "identifying with the lost object" helped me to understand how sometimes people cope with sudden loss of a beloved person by identifying with that person. Much later, I devised a simple model of the mind to explain this situation. My mind "inflated" like a balloon with anticipatory grief over Dr. Laub's anticipated death. This resulted in various symptoms such as irritability, sleeplessness, bossy behavior, etc. I coped with this "anticipated loss" by keeping him alive in my mind. So I became like him. When I finally grieved, I literally shrank my balloon, got rid of my symptoms, stopped being a brilliant psychiatrist and became my mediocre self once again.

Shortly after this incident I came to know that my wife was pregnant with our first child. Once again, I began to feel exactly like I did when Dr. Laub left for Israel. I felt irritable, angry, depressed and difficult to deal with. I remember everyone looking at me strangely, but I was powerless to stop behaving like a first class asshole. For reasons beyond me, my balloon had "inflated" again with emotions I was not aware of. One thing led to another, and the Director of Training soon targeted me, just like he targeted the dismissed American resident. He called me into his office and upbraided me for my obnoxious behavior. I broke down and let out all my pent-up emotions. He was expecting me to fight back like the American resident did. When I broke down, he was quite taken aback. He invited me to his house to comfort me. I expressed to him an overwhelming feeling of being alone, lost and unloved in a foreign country. After a good cry I told him that I felt "deflated." Somehow the word "deflated" scared him. He confessed to me his own feelings of inadequacy as the Director of Training. He recommended that I see a psychiatrist to figure out why I felt that way. I agreed if only to please the Director and prevent from being fired. Shortly thereafter, he left the hospital never to be heard of again.

I saw an elderly psychiatrist, renowned for his 'toughness,' about ten times. We talked about all and sundry but he never pegged down the issues that caused me to feel unloved, alone and abandoned. Even though the psychiatrist had great reputation, I felt that he had no clue what my problem was. I was too unaware of my inner emotions to assist him in understanding my problem. He had no clue about my issues with my parents, or my anxieties about my own future in the light of my inadequacy as a psychiatric resident. In any case, I felt a lot better just ventilating my feelings of helplessness, loneliness, and hopelessness about my future in a foreign land, and about how much I missed my family in India.

Only many years later that I realized that my becoming a prospective father had triggered resurfacing of my buried painful emotions related to my mother. My mother gave birth to three of my brothers one after another within six years of my birth. I must have felt abandoned, alone and unloved by my mother because of her preoccupation with taking care of them. As I explained in Chapter One, this was also a period when my father was very harsh on me, and I felt unloved, alone and abandoned by him also. Now, twenty-three years later, when I was about to become a father myself, the bottled-up childhood feelings of being alone, unloved and abandoned resurfaced.

Toward the end of three years at CVH, I was offered a job as a staff psychiatrist at CVH, which I accepted in principle, if only because I had not applied for another job elsewhere as yet. I had to make the choice between staying in the safe environment of CVH where my ignorance could be well hidden, and joining a new hospital, which would test my newly acquired, though very inadequate, skills. My own understanding of psychiatry was very little, and I felt very insecure. I knew one thing: if I stayed at CVH, I would be stagnating there the rest of my professional life, just as my supervisors did. I would be a frog in the dry well, totally oblivious of the great, wide and interesting world out there. All I would be doing would be drugging the unfortunate patients with antipsychotic and antidepressant drugs. I would never be able to treat the functioning people who suffered from "neurotic" symptoms on outpatient basis.

Then, to my complete surprise, I got phone calls from two eminent doctors from Yale University. Dr. Glasser, the world famous neurologist, offered me a neurology fellowship; and Dr.

Garber of Yale Child Study Center offered me fellowship under him. I had no idea what they saw in me, and fearful that I would let them both down and humiliate myself if I took up their offer, I declined. They were surprised and disappointed. They must have thought that I was a fool to decline the positions coveted by most young doctors.

The job of staff psychiatrist at CVH offered me a decent salary. However, I was willing to move elsewhere if I had a better offer. I was now a little stronger emotionally, and was willing to take a risk. Like I said, three years on this frying pan had made me "medium well." I searched for job openings in advertisements in various professional journals. Then I saw an ad that said that there were job openings for three inpatient psychiatrists in a Community Mental Health Center (CMHC) at Arden Hill Hospital, Goshen, New York. Goshen is a small town 60 miles north of New York City, known for its annual horse-trotting race. The CMHC was a 20-bed inpatient facility. The job offered a much higher salary than offered by CVH. With great trepidation I decided to apply for this job, thinking, 'no risk no gain.' I was fully prepared to be humiliated in the interview like I was during my last interview about two years earlier. But then, I had nothing to lose and everything to gain.

CHAPTER 11

Learning to Deal
with Adversity

TO ME THE LURE OF Arden Hill Hospital was purely one of remu-
neration, as I was expecting my first child, practically penniless,
sending money back home, and was still functioning in *survival
mode*. The Community Mental Health Center (CMHC) was
dedicated to taking care of acutely ill psychiatric patients in the
community. The goal was to avoid warehousing them in the State
Hospital, located at Middletown, New York. However, those patients who were dangerous to themselves or others were legally
committed there. Such patients were in the minority.

A few days after I sent in my application I received a call from
the Medical Director of the CMHC. He introduced himself as
Dr. Kenny. He gave me an appointment for the interview and
asked me to provide him with two recommendation letters from
my supervisors, which I promptly did. Both these supervisors
were from Yale University. Two weeks later I drove to Goshen, N.
Y. with my eight-month pregnant wife. Dr. Kenny, a tall, baldish

man with thin, long face and bright blue eyes, greeted me. He sized me up with his blue eyes. He was then hardly 39 years old, but he looked almost 50. He insisted that I call him Bill, adding that all staff members addressed him as Bill.

Bill repeatedly emphasized to me that his CMHC was different from all others in that, there was no hierarchy in it. The staff psychiatrist was equal in importance to all other members of the team he would be part of. There were three teams of professionals. Each team consisted of a psychiatrist, a social worker, a psychologist, a registered nurse, a licensed nurse assistant, a psychotherapist, an activity therapist, a recreational therapist, and a few other 'mental health technicians' who did the initial evaluation of patients and offered supportive therapy. In fact, Bill thought that even janitors must be considered as part of the team as they came into contact with patients on the floor.

Bill made this concept of egalitarianism in the team clear to me at the outset because he knew that many doctors harbor "God complex." He knew that many doctors from South Asia, such as India and Pakistan, suffered from "Napoleon Complex." They were almost totally unaware of the relatively less hierarchical system of America and were notorious for ordering team members around. To demonstrate to me how the system worked, Bill had set up my interview with the whole team of which I would be part of, if I were selected. He explained that he had little to do with the hiring process. The team would decide whether they wanted me as the member of their team or not. I understood this perfectly before he ushered me to the interview room.

Bill introduced me to seven or eight members of the team who were seated around a long table. Bill sat on a chair in the corner of the conference room away from the table as if to show me that he had nothing to do with the selection process. Somehow, the coolness of reception by the team members gave me a feeling that this was going to be a perfunctory interview. By my appearance alone -5'10" tall, brown skin, French-cut beard- they had made up their minds that I just did not fit into their team. For, most likely they wanted a white American doctor. Regardless, they must have decided to hold a fair trial before they hanged me.

The nurse of the team asked, "Why did you apply for this job?"

I had decided before I came for the interview that I was not going to bullshit them like most doctors do during the job interview. I was going to be true to myself, and not throw out words such as "challenge" "exciting" "love to work with people," etc. My policy has always been, 'To thine own self be true.' I never put on airs or pretended to be anyone other than myself. What you see is what you get.

"Well, I applied for this job because it pays 9,000 dollars more than the job I now have."

This statement alone must have established me as a money-hungry foreigner, or a naïve fellow who simply did not have the finesse for a proper interview.

The activity therapist, a huge lady with a bright smile, the leader of the team, asked me, "What will you contribute to our team?"

"I don't know. All I can say is that I will bring to the team whatever experience I have gained in the past three years."

The nurse asked, "What makes you think you could fit into this team?

"Well," I said, "I don't know anyone of you. How could I say how well I will fit into this team?"

The social worker said, "We have a team system here. Are you used to working with teams?"

"I have worked with teams before. Honestly, I don't know your team system. I hope I will be able to work with you all."

Obviously, my tentative answers did not impress them at all. There were no more questions from people around the table. The interview was over! They had made up their mind that I was unfit to be part of their team. The activity therapist said, "Well. Thanks for coming. We will get back with you soon."

I nodded my head and said, "Thank you." As we were all about to get up from our seats the activity therapist asked me, perhaps expecting a "No" from me, "Do you have any questions for us?"

"As a matter of fact I do," I said.

At this, all team members looked at each other and sat down. The team leader said, "Go ahead."

"Last night a curious thing happened," I said. "The telephone operator of my hospital called me to report that a drunken doctor had called her to inquire about me. Apparently he asked her what kind of a person I was. The operator asked me, 'Dr. Kamath, are you planning on leaving us?' I wondered who might have called the operator. I had already provided you with two letters of reference. I thought this call was uncalled for. It put me in an embarrassing position. I told the operator that I was going for an interview and I was not sure I would get the job. If you guys wanted more letters of reference, I would have gladly provided you with them. Whether you hire me or not makes little difference to me. I already have a job. But this phone call was certainly uncalled for. No matter, I just wanted you to know this so you would not do this to others."

The team members seemed quite taken aback by this turn of events. Obviously, the team had not expected this kind of assertiveness from a passive person like me. The team leader looked at Bill in askance. Bill's face had turned ashen. After a few tense moments Bill said, "Gee, I am sorry this happened. I had asked a colleague of mine to make discreet inquiries about you. I did not realize he would call the hospital telephone operator!" After we left the room Bill walked me to his office. There he expressed much regret for putting me through this situation. He said that the doctor who had made the call had drinking problem. I assured him that it was all right, and left.

Several days later, Bill called me and said, "The team was impressed by your assertiveness. They want you to join them. Congratulations."

I joined the Arden Hill CMHC on July 1st, 1974. The moment I attended the team meeting of team B I knew I was in serious trouble, as none of the members greeted me, nor acknowledged my presence. It was as if I did not exist. It was as if the team had concluded that I had conned them into getting this job. Or, they simply had 'buyer's remorse.' Or, they were reminding me that I should leave my M. D. degree at the door. Now I am in their territory. Perhaps the team was not comfortable dealing with a person of different racial or cultural or national background. The other two doctors hired along with me were white Americans, one an ex-military single man of Jewish faith from New York by the name of Dr. H. and the other was a white American from Boston by the name of Dr. N.

The team meeting consisted of bringing patients one by one before the team and asking them inane questions. It was obvious that the team member did not know the question's purpose. When patients did say something important, the staff missed the significance of it entirely as they were not trained to "listen." Since the team members completely ignored me, I did not actively participate in these interviews for a few days. However, when this pattern continued, I ventured to make a brief comment here and there about what the patient was trying to convey. However, the staff either did not react to my comments at all, or they sneered at it. One particularly aggressive nurse asked me, "What makes you think you are right?" Another staff said, "Why don't you just shut up and let us do our work?" I was shocked by their rudeness. Thus slapped in the face again and again, I sat at these meetings and endured the torture for two months.

I thought about leaving this job, but it was easier thought than done. My wife had given birth to our first boy exactly two weeks before I joined the CMHC, and the child was born with a serious birth defect due to the anti-emetic drug Bendectine given to my wife during pregnancy by her gynecologist.[16] I was very depressed over it myself. I had just moved to Goshen from Middletown, Connecticut. I did not want to move again with a small, sick child needing surgeries. At the same time, I did not

---

16   In spite of numerous instances of birth defects caused by this drug, Merrell Dow continued to promote this drug. Finally the drug company withdrew it in 1983. Even though a lot of people sued the company, I accepted it as my Karma and moved on. My child had to undergo 26 surgeries on his thighbone.

have the skills to deal with hostile gang of coworkers. I wondered, 'How can these people, who have so little awareness of themselves, help others?'

Bill assigned the ex-army Jewish psychiatrist Dr. H. to Team A. He was short, somewhat chubby, with fine, short curly reddish hair. He liked to suck on a lollipop like Telly Savalas did playing the role of 'Kojak' in the popular television series of the time. When he was sucking on the lollipop, Dr. H.'s identification with Kojak was obvious to all discerning people in the Center. He knew his psychiatry well and was always sure of himself. In no time at all he was able to take charge of his team and order them around. He baffled his team members by passing on to them highly technical psychiatric articles. Soon his team members were eating from his hands. Dr. H.'s fame spread around the center as someone every team must envy. He was very good with medicine. He was justifiably able to pass judgment on the treatment my patients received.

Team C's doctor was a tall baldish New Englander who looked much older than his 30 years. Dr. N. was quite the opposite in temperament from Dr. H. He was quiet and laid back. Being a white American, he did not have to suffer indignities from his equally laidback white team members. From time to time he, too, passed on an article to his team members. Dr. N. had the uncanny ability to sum up complex issues by means of simple laconic statements. His team members loved him for his qualities of quiet leadership. Shortly after I joined the center Dr. N. befriended me and introduced his lovely family to me.

I realized that Bill had assigned me to team B mainly because its members were well known in the CMHC for their aggressive and no-nonsense attitude. Perhaps he thought that I should either learn to swim quickly or drown. During the period of two months since I joined team B, members felt increasingly frustrated by the fact that I had not impressed them by passing on articles from journals. I was never in the habit of reading journals, for most of the articles had nothing to do with patient care. Research scholars wrote them, and they were often of little use to those of us who were in the trenches. By any measure, my theoretical knowledge of psychiatry was wholly inadequate. I did not know enough psychiatry to appreciate scientific articles on it. What little psychiatry I knew had to do with understanding the patient's mind. I did have the intuitive ability to understand 'psychodynamics' of patients. But I was not able to share what little I knew with the members of my team because of their uncompromising resistance to me.

Team members decided whom to admit and when to discharge patients without consulting me, even though I was legally responsible if anything went wrong. Whenever I tried to say something, one or more of team members cut me short. The whole experience with my team was frustrating as well as humiliating. This bullying went on day after day for two months. A serious crisis was bound to develop in a tense situation such as this.

During one of the evening team sessions, the dam finally burst and all the pent-up hostility of the team began to spew forth. The nurse of the team led the charge almost frothing in the mouth. She said that she was tired of me sitting like a glob in the team meeting without contributing anything to it. She told me bluntly that I should quit and go somewhere else. The social worker complained that she has learned nothing from me. A psychotherapist thumped the desk in sheer anger saying I had not passed on any articles to the team. The verbal attacks from various members continued for several minutes. During this spectacle I sat looking impassively at all my attackers. Then the attacks stopped, as if the staff expected me to say, "OK. I quit!"

"I don't think any one of you is really interested to learn psychiatry." I said quietly.

Several members shouted, "That is not true! You taught us nothing. You gave us no articles!"

"No one learns psychiatry by reading articles," I said quietly. "You learn it by listening to patients."

"But you have taught us nothing!"

"I tried to teach you many times," I said firmly. "None of you wanted to hear what I had to say. You shut me up every single time."

The crowd fell silent. Now the ball was in my court.

"You have interviewed eight patients just now. Let us review one case at a time and see what you have learned about them."

I then went around the table asking each team member questions about the patient he/she had interviewed a few minutes earlier. I asked them the hidden meaning of statements their patients made during their interviews. None of them said a word.

Then I quoted verbatim their responses and asked each of them why he/she said what he/she did. None of them answered.

"See how little you all know about your own patients?" I said quietly. "Had I been allowed to talk maybe, just maybe, we could all have learned more about the patients we are entrusted to treat."

They were all stunned for a few moments. Then one of them asked, "Where do we go from here?"

"Well. From now onwards we will discuss each patient in detail before admitting him/her, and come up with a treatment plan for that patient. No patient should be admitted or discharged without the team member discussing the case with me. Is that understood?"

All members shook their heads in agreement. There was now 'a paradigm shift' in this team system. This crisis instantly changed the dynamics of our team. By pointing out to them how their prejudices had interfered with their learning anything, I had turned the tables on them. Now I had found my proper place in the team.

This breakthrough was most welcome. The team members became my friends and we began to socialize. When the team members went out for a drink after work, they invited me to join them. For the first time since I came to America, I went out to restaurants with Americans. I threw a party to all team members at my rented duplex. They all seemed to like the Indian dishes my wife cooked for them. It looked like the team members finally accepted me as one of them. This was an entirely new experience for me, as so far I had not felt part of American life.

Within a few months later a new crisis arose. A 35-year old white woman was admitted to the acute ward with severe psychotic episode. She was extremely withdrawn and non-communicative. Stella put her forefinger in her mouth and repeated endlessly the word, "semantics." An interview with her burly husband turned up nothing. I prescribed anti-psychotic drug Thorazine by mouth for several days without any benefit. Occasionally she had to be given intramuscular injection as well.

After two weeks of unsuccessful treatment, she improved suddenly. This improvement came only after she opened up and revealed to a night staff that she had had consensual sex with a black man at work, and she carried a lot of guilt over it. Her relationship with her husband was marred by verbal and physical abuse. She was scared to tell her husband about this secret. Regardless, I did not explore this issue with Stella, as she was still rather 'brittle.' She improved with supportive therapy. Just when I felt relieved by her improvement, she presented me a new problem. She said she had throbbing pain over her left upper arm. When I inspected her arm, I saw a reddish area of about two-inch diameter. Obviously, she had developed an abscess over the area due to reaction to the Thorazine injection given to her arm by a nurse. Thorazine injections should never have been given over the arm.

I contacted a surgeon on the staff of Arden Hill Hospital. He drained the abscess. The surgery left Stella with an inch-long incision scar over her upper left arm. I discharged her with an appointment for her to see an outpatient therapist. Two weeks later, I got a phone call from the hospital administrator informing me that Stella and her husband had filed a million-dollar lawsuit against the hospital, and also against the surgeon and me individually. The couple claimed that the inch-long scar damaged its 'conjugal bliss.'

Until now I was completely oblivious about the phenomenon of frivolous lawsuits in America. This lawsuit immediately heightened all my insecurities and self-doubt even though I had nothing to do with the abscess. It was the hospital nurse who gave Stella the shot over the arm. I attended to the abscess promptly once it came to my attention. The surgeon had done his job well. To me, this was an entirely new reality of American medicine. In India, the doctor was always treated with great respect. Even if he made an honest mistake, he did not risk a lawsuit. People simply accepted bad outcome as their Karma. When lawyers of my own insurance company interviewed me, they were blatantly hostile to me. They behaved as if I had done something terribly wrong. Obviously, they were representing the insurance company, and not me. This was a thoroughly disillusioning experience for me. After a few months of mental tension, I was told that the couple settled out of court with the hospital for $ 7000. My insurance company did not have to pay out anything. Regardless, I realized that frivolous lawsuits are a way of life in America and I cannot assume that just because I gave good treatment, I would be free from lawsuits. I realized that all doctor-patient relationships are potentially adversarial. All a doctor can do is to treat the patient as well as he could and hope for the best. This was the only lawsuit by a patient I had to deal with in my 40-year long medical practice.

Arden Hill CMHC was my first real socialization experience with Americans. I was surprised how well my team members and people of other teams accepted me as one of them. A year passed in relative calm. Then Bill announced that he was promoted to the position of the Medical Director of the whole complex consisting of both inpatient and outpatient units. His office would be located in the outpatient facility next door. Dr. G., a young, dynamic, Jewish psychologist, replaced him as the Director of the inpatient unit.

Dr. G. was a stocky, red-faced bespectacled young man who was full of himself. No sooner he was appointed as the Director of the inpatient facility than he declared it as the disaster area, which he had been 'mandated' to revamp. He did not bother to meet staff members individually to know the facility's culture. He was going to be the 'hands on' guy who would take complete charge of the facility and all its activities. He reviewed every patient chart; wrote his comments and opinions on the chart; and made surprise visits to the patients at night. Clearly he was violating the boundaries separating his duties and those of doctors. He intimidated the staff and undermined their trust in the team doctors. He held all-staff meetings in which he threw dramatic temper tantrums scaring the living day light out of the staff. During one of the all-staff meeting, when he felt that the staff was not doing what he had ordered them to do, he became irate. Suddenly his face got beet red; he jumped up 6-inch high in his chair, landed on it heavily and broke its legs. Indeed, it was a scary spectacle.

Dr. G.'s behavior posed a direct threat to my mental health. Every critical note he wrote in my patients' chart could be held as evidence against me in case the patient chose to sue me for whatever reason. His perspective as a psychologist was quite different from mine as a psychiatrist. Now not only did I have to watch out for my patients, but also for my own boss. As Dr. G.'s misbehavior escalated, the staff gave in to his demands out of sheer fear. Fear psychosis gripped the entire facility. We psychiatrists on the staff also felt intimidated for reasons of our own. We dared not confront Dr. G. for fear of being fired even though it was very rare for doctors to be fired. Even self-assured Dr. H. was somewhat nonplussed. Dr. N., who normally took everything in his stride, hated Dr. G. As for me, I began to experience severe anxiety bordering on panic attacks, sleeplessness and bouts of pain in the pit of my stomach. Obviously my "balloon inflated" again due to on-going stress related to Dr. G.'s bullying. He was behaving exactly like the proverbial bull in the china shop. Years later, when my patients complained about job stress, I knew perfectly what they were talking about.

Soon, the crisis came to a head. Dr. H. led the charge against Dr. G. He began to defy Dr. G. openly. He refused to go along with Dr. G.'s orders. One thing led to another and Dr. G. decided to teach everyone who was the boss. After a heated argument with Dr. H., Dr. G. fired him from the hospital for insubordination. Dr. H. had already alienated himself from Dr. N. and me, and so we were not able to offer him much sympathy. Besides, we did not know exactly what had transpired between him and Dr. G. In any case, it was an earth-shaking event for the Center. If there was any doubt about who was in charge, Dr. H.'s firing cleared it. Everyone was scared to death wondering who would be axed next. I could not afford to lose my job, as I needed the health insurance for my sick kid, and income to support my family. Searching for another job and moving to some other hospital would take a lot of time and expense.

While all this was going on my little boy was having surgery in New York City. In addition, I had made the mistake of buying an expensive house as recommended by some of my American friends. My mindset then was such that I believed everything Americans said. I was almost totally stressed-out. This time around, my stress symptoms were very different from the ones I suffered when I was in Connecticut. I began to have mild panic attacks, and I slept fitfully at night. I am sure that these symptoms were exactly like the ones I experienced when two big bullies were kicking my butt when I was 6-9 years old. I was almost dysfunctional at work. I took a small amount of sedating antidepressant medication at night to help me sleep. I realized that I could not go on suffering like this week after week. I felt that *I must do something* to deal with this bully, come what may, or I would become very sick. None of the 60 plus employees dared to do anything for fear of meeting the same fate as Dr. H.

Mustering what little courage I had, I went to Dr. G.'s office and said, "I need to talk to you." Dr. G. asked me haughtily what it was all about. I collapsed on the chair in front of him and tried to catch my breath. Just then I saw a wilted Zebra plant on the side table in front of me. Its tall stem had bent over itself and its nearly dry leaves were hanging down touching the soil. I had seen the same plant in its lush green glory just a week before. I asked Dr. G., "I wonder what happened to that poor plant? Last week it looked so beautiful!"

Dr. G. said impatiently, "Well, last Friday evening I watered the plant but the dirt under it was so dry that water overflowed. Since I was in a rush to go home, I dug the dirt around the stem with a knife to make it absorb the water fast. I guess I cut off all the roots in the process. When I came to my office on Monday morning, the plant had wilted. I think it is now dead."

I gently slapped my forehead with my hand and exclaimed, "Oh! I should have known better than to ask you about it. That is your style!"

Suddenly Dr. G.'s face became beet-red. His eyes became tearful. He grabbed his right wrist with his left hand as if to stop his right hand from slapping me. He leaned back in his chair, took a deep breath. For a few moments he appeared stunned. After regaining his composure, he asked me, "Is that really my style?" I nodded affirmatively. "For some time now, we all in this Center have been feeling just like that Zebra plant! That was all I came to tell you." He came across like a boxer who had just received a knockout punch to the head. I did not stay there to enjoy his discomfiture. Thanking him for the meeting I left.

The problem was solved once and for all. Dr. G. was never the same again. By next day, everyone noticed a big change in his attitude as well as behavior. He seemed to be drastically "deflated" by his previous day's experience. I knew how it was to feel "deflated." He had been taken completely unawares. He was no longer so sure of himself. All this time he seemed to be belaboring under the delusion that the staff members appreciated his aggressive behavior. Obviously, he needed this "intervention." He called me aside and thanked me for saving him from the slippery slope he was on all these months. Within 24 hours after this incident I no longer had panic attacks, and I slept well without a sleeping aid. I realized the importance of solving stressful life problem creatively and as soon as possible to regain one's mental health.

Shortly after this incident, Dr. G. invited me to his house for dinner. We had a good time talking this and that. He treated me as if I was some Indian mystic. After the dinner, as I walked toward my car parked on his driveway, I heard him call me out loudly. "Bob!" As I turned my head to see why he called, waving at me he said, *"You are a better man than I am Gunga Din!"*

It was the line from Rudyard Kipling's most famous poem Gunga Din (1892). The poem is a rhyming narrative from the point of view of a British soldier about an Indian water bearer (bhisti) who dies while saving the soldier's life. Like several of Kipling's poems, Gunga Din extoled the virtues of a humble Indian while revealing the racism of a colonial infantryman who viewed him as being of "lower order." The poem is best known for its oft-quoted last stanza: *"Tho' I've belted you and flayed you, by the livin' Gawd that made you, you're a better man than I am, Gunga Din."* The poem was published as one of the martial poems called the Barrack-Room Ballads. (Check Google).

Soon a new problem cropped up. A social worker in my team who worked mostly at night continued to harbor hateful feelings toward me for no valid reason other than he simply did not like foreigners. Bob worked mostly in the evening shift when I was not around. That gave him plenty of opportunity to sabotage any treatment my patients got from me. I noticed a curious phenomenon with my patients. Many of them turned hostile to me whenever I interviewed them in the morning. They questioned me regarding the medications I prescribed them, or they did not agree with anything I said about their problems. It became increasingly clear to me that Bob and a small coterie of his cohorts undermined at night everything I was doing during the daytime.

One day Bob announced that he was recruiting a night nurse to replace the one who left the hospital. He picked a forty-year old male nurse to join our team for the night shift. Of course, he did not bother to consult about this appointment with Dr. M or me. The male nurse came to work at night and left the hospital before we came to work, and so I never had a chance to meet with him. Within one month after his appointment, a female patient filed a complaint that he had entered her room at night and molested her. This created a major problem for our team as well as the hospital. Following the internal investigation, the male nurse was fired. As it turned out, the male nurse had history of molesting patients, and Bob knew it when he hired him. During one of morning team meetings, I confronted Bob with the fact that he had hired the male nurse knowing full well his problem at his previous jobs. I told him, "Bob, just so you can get back at me, you didn't mind at all risking the safety of our patients, right?" Bob had no defense. When I shared this anecdote with a psychiatrist friend of mine, he asked me a question, "Do you know what the difference is between psychiatric patients and the staff?" I said, "No." he replied dryly, "Well, psychiatric patients always get better!"

During my work with staff of other hospitals, I confirmed what I had realized at Arden Hill Hospital CMHC. It is not enough if the psychiatrist overcomes the natural psychological resistance of patients in revealing themselves, he must first deal with the resistance of the staff members as well. Staff members often forget that they must set aside their prejudices and hatred and focus on the welfare of the patients. Very often people with serious personal issues seek employment in psychiatric facilities as a way of dealing with them. They act out their issues with patients as well as doctors.

Over the years I found out how difficult it is to provide psychiatric care for even my private clients. For every single effort I put in to get my patients well, there were at least one half-dozen people around them who attempted to sabotage it. Invariably, my patients got unsolicited or solicited advice from well-meaning relatives, friends, pastors, nurses, doctors, and others, which undermined just about everything I said or did to get them well. Various talk shows further contributed to this problem. To minimize this, I gave my patients a pamphlet telling them not to listen to others' advice, including what they heard on popular talk shows. Sabotage of treatment by family members is more common than most psychiatrists realize. I wrote in the pamphlet, "If you want to listen to other's advice regarding your treatment, you don't need me."

There were numerous interesting incidents at this CMHC, but space does not permit me to share most of them. Here is one such incident: On one occasion an 18-year old white woman was brought to the hospital by her family in a state of catatonic stupor. In this disorder, the patient becomes extremely withdrawn, uncommunicative and assumes stiff, statue-like body posture. In this state of mind, it was impossible to obtain any information from her. In cases such as this, the main treatment is to give patient anti-psychotic drugs to control the symptoms.

The staff presenting this case to me was a 30-year old nurse who had joined our team just a few weeks earlier. I asked her, "Well, what do you think is happening with his girl?" She was too inexperienced to answer my question. Pointing my forefinger at the ceiling over the head of the patient I asked her, "What do you see hanging over there?" She looked up at the ceiling and said, "I see nothing!" I said, "Don't you see a sword hanging over the head of this poor girl?" Confused by this silly conversation, she said, "I don't get it. What do you mean?"

"Have you heard of the sword of Damocles?" I asked her.

"Yes," she said.

"You see reaction like this in people who are scared to death that something terrible is going to happen to them. They are trapped in some really bad life situation from which they cannot escape. So they freeze. Often they have helpless rage within them which is ready to explode."

With drug treatment and supportive therapy the patient improved within two weeks. As it turned out, this patient's stepfather was sexually abusing her. Our theory turned out to be right, at least in this case. Unfortunately, this incident led to some unintended consequences. A few days later the nurse showed up at my office and said she wanted to talk with me. I asked her to sit down. She said that she had a crush on me. I was shocked by this development. She went on to tell me that she had never met anyone like me before; no one ever taught her anything like I did; and she had learned more about human behavior from me than anyone else. Now she could not get me out of her mind.

This kind of infatuation of female staff with male authority figure is common. I was at a loss for words. I said to myself, "What a jam I have gotten myself into!" I told her, "Listen. I am sorry if I gave you a wrong impression. I am a married man. I was merely teaching you psychiatry in a way that would make you think. There was nothing more to it." She was very disappointed and hurt. She left my office in tears. Now I faced a new dilemma. Should I keep this encounter a secret, or should I reveal it to my teammates. The danger in not exposing this to my teammates lay in the fact that she might act out her anger leading to disruption of patient care and unnecessary rumors. During the next team meeting, I told my team members what had happened and explained the reason for my sharing this information with them. I told them that exposing this situation at this stage itself was safer than after complications had developed. They all agreed.

The next day the angry nurse showed up at my office and said to me, "I wish you had not told other team members what happened. You are a coward!" She stormed out of my office. This incident taught me an important lesson. Many staff members might try to fulfill their repressed unmet needs and wants through their relationship with me. I should be more careful how I behaved with them. Later on when couple of other female staff members showed inordinate interest in me, I began to tone down the intensity of my interaction with them.

Three highly eventful years passed like this. My exposure to real Americans gave me the confidence that I was ready for a more challenging job. I had better handle on my profession, and I had better skill in dealing with the staff. I appeared for Part One of American Board of Psychiatry and Neurology and passed. It was time to move on in search of a more challenging job. I started looking for a position of Medical Director of a CMHC in the heartland of America.

An advertisement in The Psychiatric News caught my eyes. The ad said that St. Francis Medical Center in Cape Girardeau,

Missouri, was looking for a full time Medical Director for its newly expanded facility. I looked up on the map where Missouri was. It was so far from New York! When I asked my friends about it they said, "Oh, my! That is a godforsaken place. People over there don't like colored people." But I was ready to move on. I felt confident that I could handle this job well. On a 8x5 inch paper I handwrote the as follows:

Dear. Dr. Lebedun,

I am writing this in response to your ad in The Psychiatric News seeking a Medical Director for your CMHC. I am currently employed as the staff psychiatrist at CMHC at Goshen, N. Y. I received my psychiatric train-ing in the Yale University affiliated program at Connecticut Valley Hospital, Middletown, CT. I have passed Part One of Psychiatric Board Exam. I want you to know that I am very dark-skinned. If this poses a problem, please ignore this letter. I do understand.
Sincerely,
K. P. S. Kamath, M. D.

I did not expect a response. But I was in for a pleasant surprise.

CHAPTER 12
New Kid in Town

Two days later, I got a phone call from Dr. Lebedun's Administrative Assistant (AA). She said that the Administrative Director Dr. Lebedun would like for me to fly down to Cape Girardeau, Missouri for an interview. I had not expected such a quick response. I was used to not being wanted anywhere. I had sent the letter just to test the waters. I tried to buy time by saying, "Let me think about it."

Yolanda called me back later that day. "We need you to come for the interview as soon as possible. I will send you the ticket for your flight."

"Well" I said. "I cannot accept your air ticket. I do not like to be under anyone's obligation."

This took Yolanda aback. She was used to candidates asking her to send money for airfare, hotel, etc. The ticket to Cape Girardeau was expensive, but I wanted to reserve my right to decline any offer without feeling that I had taken advantage of the hospital's largess. I flew to Cape Girardeau, MO via Memphis, TN. Dr. Dr. Lebedun came to receive me at the tiny airport of Cape Girardeau. He was a thinly built man with salt and pepper kinky hair. He was very pleasant. He said that the Community Mental Health Center at St. Francis Medical Center was being expanded. Up till then, they had a part time psychiatrist to take care of their outpatient as well as inpatients. He was not happy that the doctor was not available most of the time because of his commitment to his private practice. The Center was hiring two full time doctors, one for inpatient and one for outpatient. If hired, I would be the Medical Director in charge of the whole facility but working mostly with very sick inpatient population.

Dr. Lebedun showed me a pile of 97 applications for the job from all over the country. Some of them had attached their pay-check stubs to the application to show how much they were earning already, and how much they expected in salary and night calls. Some resumes were ten-pages long. I saw my 8x5 inch hand-written letter on the top of the heap. He said, "Everyone wants to know how much we paid for this or that. Everyone wants me to send him airline ticket. You are the only one who made no financial demands. I don't care how dark-skinned you are. Bob, we need you here."

Obviously, I was no longer functioning on *survival mode*. Now, I wanted to test my newly gained confidence by accepting a truly challenging job. Now I wanted to be in charge of my life as well as my practice.

"Well, let me think about it for a day or two," I said. At this, Dr. Lebedun offered me 4,000-dollar increase in the salary to induce me to join the staff. I said, "You must know by now that money is not the issue here. I need to discuss this with my wife."

The day after I returned home, Dr. Lebedun called me saying, "Bob, we need you here, real bad." Even though my wife was a little hesitant, I convinced her that we are ready for new adventure in the Heartland of America. However, I told Dr. Lebedun that I would be available only for two years as I planned to return to India after that "to do some fundamental work there." He agreed to my terms on condition that I would keep it a secret. He wanted me to fly over again to attend a cocktail party to introduce me to the 37-member medical staff.[17] This time around, he insisted on reimbursing me the cost of both flights. I flew again to Cape and met all the doctors of the city. Those days, foreign trained doctors were still a curiosity. I was received with open arms. I had never felt more welcome in America.

Back in Goshen, I submitted my resignation to my position and prepared to move to Missouri. I put my house for sale and left for Missouri by car with my wife and three year old son. I reached Cape Girardeau on September 7th, 1977. Crossing the rickety bridge over the Mississippi River from IL shortly after sunset, the city of Cape Girardeau looked beautiful on the Missouri side. As I crossed the bridge I turned the radio on. I was amused to hear Eagle's song "New Kid in Town" was playing… "Everybody loves you, don't let them down!"

I had rented a two-bedroom apartment near the hospital. When I checked in, the supervisor came to orient me to the place. Noting that I was a colored person, he said, "We don't like loud music and wild parties over here." I assured him that I understood perfectly what he meant. Two days later the local newspaper

---

17 Today there are about 300 physicians in Cape Girardeau, MO.

showed an 8X 6-inch picture of me on the front page announcing that I would be the new Medical Director of St. Francis Mental Health Center. When the supervisor saw this, he came to me to inquire how I was doing and if there was anything he could do to make our stay comfortable. It was obvious that he was somewhat embarrassed by the way he treated me two days earlier.

The team I was to work with was far more cohesive and accepting than the one I encountered in New York. Having dealt with New York attack dogs these people came across as pussy-cats. They were anxious to learn. They cooperated with me to the fullest extent. No sooner was the inpatient unit expanded, than patients began to show up for admission. Soon I was busy taking care of acutely ill people who came for disorders ranging from psychosis to depression. Dr. Lebedun hired new staff to meet the expanding needs. And the hospital made a lot of money from the inpatient revenue.

A 57-year old female psychiatrist, who was extremely dedicated to her patients, staffed the outpatient department. Her devotion to her patients was so great that she always neglected her paper work. No matter how dedicated one is to the patient care, documentation is essential. Dr. Lebedun often complained with me that Dr. L. was behind in her paperwork, which had resulted in problems with billing. The point was that billing was at the very top of all priorities when it came to survival of the Center. He wanted me to intervene, as his requests had fallen on deaf ears. When I approached Dr. L. very gently about this chronic problem, she became very upset. Apparently her late husband was a victim of Hitler's concentration camps in Poland. My gentle prodding seemed to have reminded her of her husband's Nazi tormentors. I never said anything to hurt her feelings, but she was obviously looking at me through the tinted glasses. This is an example of how our past traumatic issues stay with us every single moment, and color everything we see around us.

When a doctor does good work, he would get more referrals. It was not possible to say no to referring doctors without losing their goodwill. To ensure the quality of care, I went to the hospital in the middle of the night for admission even though I could have waited till the morning. The hospital's fame spread wide, I got more referrals. The hospital made a lot of money. As our patient load increased, I had to work 16 hours a day, and soon I felt totally overwhelmed by the workload. Soon the wear and tear of the job began to show. I developed stomach ulcers. A gastroenterologist diagnosed me as suffering from gastro-esophageal reflux and stomach ulcer. I had to start taking antacids. I talked with Dr. Lebedun about the possibility of hiring another psychiatrist. He was not happy with this. His solution was that I should slow down and not do such a good job! I asked him, "How could I reduce the quality of work I am doing?" After failing in several tries, I told him that I was ready to quit. He was mortified.

Soon the center began the search for a new psychiatrist. After interviewing a few candidates, Dr. Lebedun and I settled for a tall, bearded Englishman. Dr. B. was a highly learned psychiatrist who read a lot of psychiatric journals. However, he had somewhat limited knowledge of psychodynamics –knowledge of what made people tick. His patients liked his British accent, but in the end, they did not know what exactly he said about their problems. He was good with his medicine, a reflection of how psychiatry had already begun to drift in the direction of becoming a "medical specialty." During those days psychiatrists were desperately trying to become "medical specialists." Psychodynamics had begun to take back seat to drug treatment.

I shifted my office to the outpatient department and began to see some functioning patients with depression and anxiety. Even though I was not too good at figuring out psychodynamics of outpatients, I intuitively knew what ticked my patients. The proof of this came in the form of increased referrals and letters from referring doctors. Here is a quote from a letter by a local family physician dated July 30, 1979:

> *Dear Dr. Kamath,*
> *I wish to express my appreciation for the follow-up information given the patients that are referred to you. I cannot remember ever receiving a letter from another doctor giving as much useful information about a patient as the recent one I received concerning Mrs. So and So. I am sure she is receiving the very best of care. She certainly had a very thorough evaluation as indicated in your note. I am glad that you are continuing to see this woman and have every reason to believe that you can help.*
> *Sincerely yours,*
> *M. E. C. M.D.*

Such goodwill I created was a greater reward than any money I could have made from this job. For, when I established my own private practice in Cape Girardeau in August 1982, all these doctors supported me by sending a steady stream of patients. They were paying me back for the assistance I had given them in managing their patients three years earlier.

During my two-years and three months of employment at CMHC, I saw many interesting cases. But I learned more than ever before the power of kindness in healing patients in distress. A middle-aged woman, mother of two girls admitted her 16-year old daughter to the psychiatric unit. She said the daughter was always angry and acting out. The mother said that she had lost a lot of sleep over her daughter's behavior. The pediatrician referred her to me saying, "If someone can help you, it is Dr. Kamath."

The patient was a pretty teenager who was angry that her parents were not getting along. She grew up seeing her parents fight all the time. Obviously, the girl was precipitating a crisis to resolve her parent's problems one way or another. The mother came across as very distraught, exhausted and hopeless. After my session with the patient, I met with the mother and reassured her that her daughter would be all right, and that her acting out was more due to her love for her than hate. I told her that in her old age this very daughter would be there by her side. The mother felt very reassured. I accompanied her to the stairs to see her off. At that moment, overwhelmed by her relief, she began to faint. I grabbed her arm and asked, "Are you all right?" She looked very pale. Instinctively I said, "Do you want me to carry you down the stairs?"

The mother looked at me incredulously. Obviously, my spontaneous kindness touched her deeply. After she recovered, and I accompanied her down the stairs and to her car. The next day she called me to say that she slept the best in years. She felt completely well knowing that her daughter was in safe hands. With counseling, the daughter got well. The mother divorced her husband and moved to Florida. She kept in touch with me till her death 30 years later.

A young man came to see me for recurrent panic attacks. He did not know why. In the interview he revealed that within a couple of years after his marriage, his wife divorced him. He was deeply hurt. He felt like a failure. He ventilated his feelings of inadequacy, shame and guilt. After a couple of sessions, I told him, "It takes two to tango. You are only 50% responsible for this divorce. Now that you have dealt with these painful emotions, you should move on with life. You will not have another panic attack, I assure you." The young man never had another panic attack. He went on to become a famous person in this area.

Several judges in the city befriended me and asked me to give my professional opinion in resolving difficult cases. A judge wrote, "Your help and interest in some very difficult cases always made the difference in reaching the right decision for a particular patient." Local lawyers consulted me frequently regarding their cases. I was invited to speak to various local organizations. During my employment at St. Francis CMHC, I became more confident both as a psychiatrist and as a person. I felt completely in charge of my life and profession. I had come a long way since the dark days of 1970. The hospital validated my usefulness by giving me generous raises in salary even without my asking. I mingled with more Americans and became somewhat 'Americanized.' These were the best years for me in America thus far.

In spite of all this, I had no plans to settle down in America. In Chapter One I discussed how an old traumatic emotional issue resurfaced in 1975, and how I became obsessed with returning to India to do "some fundamental work there." I wanted to go back to India and be part of nation-building effort. I knew well that returning to India was more daunting than anything I had faced in the United States. However, my experience as the Medical Director of St. Francis Mental Health Center prepared me very well for this formidable task.

Exactly two years after I joined the hospital, I announced that I would be leaving for India in December 1979. It sent shock waves in the Center. For, the staff were not used to working with doctors who cared for their patients as I did. An elderly nurse I had worked with had moved to Texas a few months earlier. When she heard the news, she wrote me this poignant letter dated September 19, 1979, which I have cherished to this day:

Dear Bob,

Really I meant to write you a note shortly after leaving St. Francis. I think I put it off for fear of sounding somewhat maudlin. Recently I had a letter from Betty Meyer in which she said you planned to return to India. So what I have to say had better be said before you leave the country. And put briefly that something is simply —you are the greatest! I'll never forget what I learned from you and as is usually the case, actions speak louder than words. I will remember

your examples of kindness, concern and true empathy. The one American whom I would compare you is Robert Coles, Professor of Psychiatry and Medical Humanities at Harvard Medical School. America can ill afford to lose you, but I daresay India needs you more. I shall look forward to seeing your name on at least one book in years to come.
All good wishes,
Liz B.

On October 12th, Dr. Lebedun held a meeting with all staff members and asked me to give them the principles by which a CMHC must abide by in offering the public their service. He summarized what I said in a note he sent to all of them on December 16th:

At our get-together on October 12, Dr. Kamath expressed briefly and well goals, which I believe are valuable to the proper working of our program. Here they are for your review.

1. *Operate as an institution with a public conscience and the efficiency of a private concern.*
2. *Project a "good people" image to the community.*
3. *Be relevant to the community by identifying its needs and meeting them.*
4. *Personalize your dealings with people —people trust individuals, not institutions.*
5. *Let "patient care" be your primary preoccupation all the time.*
6. *Recognize the "buck stops here" —we are here to be used.*

7.   *Be aware always of "process" and "responsibility."*

8.   *Give more than you take… Growth comes only through hard work and sacrifice.*

9.   *Avoid, at all cost, conflict with the patient. You will lose when conflict occurs.*

10. *When dealing with the public, let us not have an attitude of being "experts." We are here to serve them and no one should be refused help because she/he doesn't know how to ask for it.*

Dr. Lebedun gave me a plaque, which appreciated me *"For outstanding leadership as a Medical Director of the Community Mental Health Center, and for directing, achieving and maintaining the highest standard of excellence in the delivery of mental health services for all who came to St. Francis Medical Center for their care. Signed: Board of Directors, St. Francis Medical Center.*

Suffice it to say that by December 1979, I was ready to move to India. My boys were five and one year old. My wife was almost always in tears about this decision. But I could not resist my urge. I had to resolve some childhood traumatic issues to redeem myself.

When finally the time came for me to say goodbye, both the staff and I were very sad. On December 15th, 1979, I packed everything in my car and drove off to New York crossing Mississippi River over the same rickety bridge I had crossed 27 months earlier. When I turned the radio on. Robert John's song "Sad Eyes" played on every station I tuned: *"Looks like it's over, you knew I couldn't stay. We had a good thing, I miss your sweet love… It's* over... Sad eyes, turn the other way, I don't wanna see you cry. Sad eyes, you knew there would come a day when we would have to say 'goodbye.'

CHAPTER 13

Cleaning the Augean Stables

IN CHAPTER ONE I EXPLAINED how I redeemed myself through 18-month long struggle against institutionalize corruption and injustice in India. By the end of 18 months of my stay in India, however, I had spent all my savings in the service of India, and I was practically penniless. I was ready to return to America, though temporarily. I needed to go back to America, make some money and return home to continue to fight corruption. My psychiatric practice in India had not done well, as the stigma of psychiatric disorders was very strong, and my income was not enough to support my family. Small town India was not ready for a psychiatrist.

In the 3rd week of April 1981, I received a letter from Fred M., the Superintendent of Farmington State Hospital at Farmington, Missouri. Apparently Fred was looking for a Chief of Staff for the State Hospital, even if it was for a short period of time. Farmington State Hospital was in dire straights. The hospital had lost Medicare Certification three years in a row. If it did not regain certification in its fourth attempt, it would stop receiving Federal money for the care of Medicare patients. It was rumored that the State of Missouri was planning to close the hospital down due to poor patient care. Many doctors on the staff were drug addicts or alcoholics. About one thousand jobs were in jeopardy.

This letter was fortuitous. Even though the salary offered by quite a bit less than what I was making in Cape Girardeau, I accepted his offer on condition that that would be a one-year assignment. I left for America on May 14th 1981. When I landed in St. Louis, Neil Diamond's song "They come to America, Today!" was on the intercom: *Far, we've been traveling far, without a home but not without a star… on the boat and on the planes they come to America, never looking back… They come to America!"* How apt, I thought. I did not know then that circumstances would force me to stay in America the rest of my life.

This was the first time I had been to the godforsaken Farmington State Hospital. Separating the hospital premise from the road was a high rocky wall, which reminded me of a prison. As I entered the premise through the wide opening in the wall, I saw in front of me a wide tree-lined road leading to an impressive 19th century limestone building a furlong ahead. I saw on left the side three-story high brick buildings located on well-manicured lawns. Zombie-like patients loitered here and there in a daze.

Fred received me cordially and briefed me about the arduous task ahead. First thing he told me was that the non-medical staff had some questions to ask me, as they had been offended by some critical comments about the hospital I made when I was the Medical Director of St. Francis Mental Health Center two years earlier. I had, indeed expressed my irritation at the complacent Farmington staff for the bureaucratic hurdles they threw at people who tried to get help there. The bitter truth is that government-run hospitals are basically there for the employment of the staff. The second thing he wanted me to do was to find whatever excuse I could to fire a cantankerous internist on the staff, who had been a thorn on his side for many years. Fred and Dr. T. hated each other passionately. Third assignment he gave me was to hire new psychiatrists to raise the standard of patient care, and get rid of doctors with chemical dependency problems. Obviously, Fred had given me the Herculean task of cleaning the Augean Stables of a lot of horseshit that had accumulated over the past few decades.

The hospital offered me a nice house on the campus to live in. At the earliest opportunity, I met with the entire non-medical staff to resolve their resentments about my critical comments of the past. I admitted to having made critical remarks about the way the hospital handled the admission process and explained the helplessness felt by the general public regarding the hospital's admission policies and procedures. I told the staff that a taxpayer-funded hospital such as this must develop an attitude of helpfulness. After the staff ventilated their displeasure about my comments, the meeting was over. We all made up and there were no unresolved issues left. The fact of the matter was that they needed me so badly that they had to simply set aside their personal grievance and move on with the task of saving the hospital from closure. A social worker that was a fixture of the hospital for over thirty years kept telling again and again, "I am a survivor."

Obviously he was scared that I might fire him. I had no power to fire anyone. I felt nothing but compassion for them as well as all the medical staff working there.

Next I met with the medical staff. There were eight staff physicians on board two of whom were internists. The remaining five were non-Board certified psychiatrists. All of them appeared to be extremely anxious not knowing what to expect from me. Every psychiatrist was afraid of being fired by me, not knowing that I had compassion for their situation and had no intention of getting rid of them. My best bet was to work with them to get the best out of them. One of the psychiatrists was a 55-year old alcoholic who came to the meeting drunk. Another was a 60-year old polish psychiatrist who was extremely insecure as evidenced by his tearfulness whenever he opened his mouth. Then there was a young Eastern European female psychiatrist, who talked a lot as a way of covering up her fear. She had little ability to listen to anyone around her. Of the two internists, one was a tall American who spoke extremely slowly, and was fairly comfortable with his own state of affairs. The other was Dr. T., a grey haired dour man in his early sixties wearing thick horn-rimmed eyeglasses. This was the internist Fred was anxious to get rid of as soon as possible.

Dr. T. was a fairly competent internist whose main claim to his usefulness was that he could read EKG. On the negative side, he was always ill tempered, intimidating of the staff, and not easy to work with. He often spoke ill of Fred and threatened to sue the hospital if he was ever fired. He often blackmailed Fred and missed no opportunity to threaten to bring the "whole goddamn hospital down with me." Apparently he had some dark secrets of the hospital with him, which he was not hesitant to reveal to the newspapers and televisions. Over the course of next few weeks, Fred kept asking me when I would fire him, to which I always replied, "We can't fire him unless he has done something terribly wrong. We can't be unjust about it no matter how cantankerous this guy might be."

I had more urgent matters to attend to. The acute care psychiatric wards were filled with acutely ill patients who had been committed there for being dangerous to themselves or others. Within 72 hours after their admissions I had to evaluate them and decide if they needed to be recommitted or released. They needed to be treated for whatever their psychiatric disorders were. The acute care wards were nothing short of bedlam. Psychotic patients ran wildly in the corridors chased by the frantic staff. Some of them were restrained to protect other residents.

The first thing I did was to call a meeting of all male patients in the Receiving Hall. I sat with them in a circle. This was something new to patients as well as the staff. It became apparent to all of them that now there was someone in charge, who was willing to listen to them. I went around the circle inquiring about everyone's problems. Psychotic patients said nothing, being preoccupied with their own inner thoughts. Others ventilated their frustrations openly. Soon patients began to look forward to these meetings. Within a month after I took over, the wards were pacified and order was restored.

Aside from diagnosing accurately the newly admitted patients and treating them with proper medications, my task consisted of reevaluate patients who had been recommitted there for longer stay. Many of these patients suffering from Bipolar disorder, then known as Manic-Depressive disorder, had been misdiagnosed as Schizophrenic and were on large doses of potent antipsychotic medications. Once they were put on Lithium, a wonderful mood stabilizer, they got well and were discharged promptly. All this took long hours of work and diligent review of patients' records.

The State of Missouri had mandated that State Hospitals should no longer serve as warehouses for chronically ill people. FSH used to warehouse over a thousand inpatients till recently. The mandate required that most of these patients be placed in halfway houses and boarding homes in the community. It was my responsibility to review their records and dismiss them from the hospital. This meant closing down of many age-old wards and letting go of staff that had worked there for decades. I could see how the staff was very nervous about losing their jobs. I was perceived at once as a savior of the hospital and at once as a destroyer of staff's jobs. Those who felt secure about their jobs supported my work; those who feared losing their jobs were clearly not happy with me. However, when they saw me showing up for admission in the middle of the night, spend long hours interviewing patients whom no one cared to talk with, they seemed to have been impressed by my dedication. Gradually, I sensed a good deal of respect from all staff members.

In the course of my work at FSH hospital, the reality that hospitals serve as an important source of jobs for the community dawned on me more forcefully than ever. The employees of the hospital have unconscious need to keep the hospital filled with patients to keep their jobs secure. Any attempt to empty the hospital risked their livelihood. I have found this to be true during my stint at other institutions as well. The staff's primary concern is their own jobs, not the welfare of patients. Unconsciously, they sabotaged any attempt to empty the beds.

During the review of charts of patients who had been at FSH for over twenty years I came across the chart of one David C., a thirty six year old white man who had been admitted there for the first time at age 16. His mother committed him there because she could not handle him at home. The main complaint was that he smoked pot. Subsequently, he had been released and re-hospitalized numerous times for "violent behavior." After a few years, David was routinely re-committed to the hospital even without discharge. He became a permanent fixture on one of the wards. I interviewed David and found out that there was absolutely no reason for David to be in the hospital. David expressed much desire to leave the hospital and be in a halfway house. So I prepared the needed legal papers for his release; got an appointment for a hearing at the county court in Benton, MO, and drove there with David for a hearing. There I testified to the judge that David no longer needed to be in the hospital. The judge granted his release immediately. I drove back to the hospital, dropped him back in front of his dormitory and drove straight to my home just one minute away.

The phone was ringing as I entered my home. When I answered, the voice on the other end said, "Dr. Kamath, you better come over right away. David broke the arm of our social worker. He is in a straight jacket. We can't have him here anymore. He should be shipped to Fulton State Maximum Security." I rushed back to David's ward. When I entered it, David was in a straight jacket, sitting on the floor. A few staff members surrounded him as if they were ready to pounce on him if he moved even a little.

"David, what happened," I asked.

"After you dropped me off, I entered the building. The social worker and one of the staff stood on either side of the door. As I passed between them, they said 'Faggot!' and I said 'You are faggots, not me.' They both pushed me and I pushed them back. The social worker fell and broke his arm. I didn't hit him."

I knew the social worker well. He was an alcoholic man in his late fifties. He was very emaciated due to alcoholism. I came to know later that he suffered from osteoporosis. In any case, his right arm bone broke at the shoulder and he had to be hospitalized. The staff was adamant that David was a dangerous person and he must be sent to Fulton. They were bent on teaching both David and me a lesson. I had no choice but to sign papers to ship David to Fulton for I knew for sure that had I not done that, David's life would be in danger.

From then onwards, every year for nearly ten years I received a letter from David begging me to do something to liberate him from the jaws of state sponsored injustice. I was helpless to do anything, as now David provided job security to the staff of Fulton State Hospital. I lost touch with David in due course.

I recruited a new psychiatrist who appeared to be conscientious and hardworking. Once he came on board, I felt more confident in asking better performance from other psychiatrists. On one occasion, Dr. M., a psychiatrist, did not show up for work. I went to his cottage on the hospital premise to see what was happening. The front door was open. When I entered the house, I was shocked to find it in great deal of disarray. As I entered the living room, I saw Dr. M. on the floor. At first I thought he was dead. When I called out his name, he moved. He was extremely drunk. He had not shaved in several days. He was half naked. There was urine and feces all over the floor. With the help of a couple of staff, I had him cleaned up. I made arrangement for his admission to a local hospital. He never returned to work. Two more psychiatrists, who were providing no care or poor care, were also retired. The burden of caring for their patients fell on me. Sometimes I was taking care of several hundred psychiatric patients.

One Friday evening I got a call from one of the wards that an elderly woman had slipped into coma. She had fallen down that afternoon and hurt her head. Dr. T. had examined her and found nothing to worry about. He had left the hospital for the weekend and that is why they had called me. I went to the ward and found the patient in coma. She was bleeding in the brain. I arranged for her admission to Barnes Hospital at St. Louis.

Two days later I received a call from Barnes Hospital that the patient died from brain hemorrhage. Fred saw his chance to get rid of Dr. T. He came to me saying, "Bob. I think this is our chance to fire this SOB." I told him that this was an innocent mistake on the part of Dr. T. This could have happened to even me. I asked him to be patient.

Dr. T. must have expected that I was going to fire him any time now. He went around telling the staff that he was not going to let "this two bit Hindoo fire me." I just let things take their course. Soon complaints about Dr. T. began to pour in. Nurses said that he had become more irritable than ever before. He yelled at the staff. It was impossible to have any meaningful interaction with him. Obviously, his balloon was ready to pop! The chief nurse wanted to have a staff meeting with him to confront him with his behavior. She wanted me in that meeting. I agreed to attend the meeting.

In the meeting that followed, ten staff members showed up. Dr. T. appeared very nervous. The chief nurse explained to him the purpose of that meeting. At this, Dr. T. became very upset and tearful, and said, "I am out of here." He left the meeting abruptly.

That evening I received a phone call from Dr. T. at my home. He was very angry. He said, "Listen to me Dr. Kamath. If you think that you can fire me, you better think again. I can create a lot of trouble for you!"

I said politely, "Dr. T., I don't know what you are talking about. I have no plans to fire you. You have been a great asset to FSH. Why don't you come over for a glass of beer? Let's talk it over." Reassured, he agreed. We sat down and had a good talk over cold beer. I told him that we had no plans to fire him. "In fact," I told him, "without you, who will take care of all these patients? Who will read EKGs?"

"Fred wants me out. I have known that for a long time. But let me tell you this: If the SOB fires me, I will go to newspapers and expose all the dirty secrets of this goddamn hospital. They will close this goddamn place tomorrow."

"What terrible secrets are you talking about, Dr. T.?"

"I can give you long laundry list. The staff stealing drugs meant for patients, for one thing."

"Dr. T., this hospital is already in such a bad shape that nothing you reveal would make things any worse for it. You know well that I was hired to clean the accumulated horseshit of Augean Stables of this goddamned hospital. If newspapers and television reporters ask me whether your allegations are true, I will tell them to believe every single word you told them! I will tell them that I was hired to clean up the mess you were talking about."

Dr. T. was not prepared for my nonchalance. He said, "Well, I would like to quit my job. I just can't stand it anymore. I want to resign from my job."

"I think you are making a big mistake. Please reconsider your decision."

"No. I must go. I must tell you though that if Fred badmouths me and makes it hard for me to get a job elsewhere, I will sue the shit out of him."

"I know how you feel about Fred. I assure you he will do nothing of that sort. Since you insist on retiring, I would like to give you a great recommendation letter so that you can get a job anywhere you apply. Let us meet at Fred's office at eight O'clock tomorrow morning. You can handover your resignation letter to him then."

The next morning, we went to Fred's office. I told him that Dr. T. had resigned and I had reluctantly accepted his resignation. I asked him to assure Dr. T. that he would not say anything bad about him to anyone. Fred gave verbal assurances to Dr. T. I handed over my recommendation letter to Dr. T. We shook hands and parted ways.

My next challenge was to get the Medicare recertification for the hospital without which the hospital would be closed in three months. The Assistant Superintendent was a highly competent woman by the name of Fanny Lou, who was in her fifties. She was a typical bureaucrat who admonished all incompetent staff by her usual epithet, "concern." This word meant that the person had not done his or her job right. Everyone talked about her as someone addicted to alcohol, but I never smelled it on her breath. She smoked incessantly, while poring over her files. I worked closely with her to prepare for the Medicare team inspection.

I was supposed to have a By-laws folder ready for the Medicare team but not being a bureaucrat, I just could not bring myself to writing it. The Chief of Staff of St. Louis State Hospital came down to Farmington and showed me a two-inch thick folder of By-laws. When I told him that I did not have this document to show, he said, "You can't get certification without this document." But it was too late for me to create this folder. Besides I was up to my arse in the swamp looking after my sick patients. Instead I prepared myself to answer verbally any and all questions the Medicare team might have for me.

Finally the dreaded day of Medicare inspection arrived. I was ushered into the office of the Superintendent to be introduced to Dr. W., the Medicare team leader. He had now occupied Fred's chair. As Dr. W. went over my Curriculum Vitae, he suddenly looked up in amazement and said, "You trained at Connecticut Valley! I was the assistant Superintendent of CVH just before you joined! It is a small world!" Obviously, he did not know about my low opinion about CVH, and how I was responsible for it losing

JCAH license. We made instant *emotional connection*. From that moment onwards I could do no wrong. As I walked with him and his team members from building to building, I explained to him various steps I had taken to raise the standard of medical care. I went over with him my recruitment efforts; changes in hospital policies in caring for the very sick, so on and so forth. On one occasion, before he could point out to me a stain on a ceiling, I pointed my finger at it and said that the order for repair of that roof above it has already been sent.

Normally, tons of documents would be needed to pass Medicare Certification visit such as this. We presented no written records. We just talked the whole Medicare team through hundreds of improvements that had already been implemented and hundreds more that would be. By the end of two days, the team was rather pleased. The Medicare team recertified the hospital. Fred threw a big party for the team and the staff I received a glowing letter of appreciation from the Director of Mental Health Department of the State of Missouri. Shortly thereafter, the Governor approved five million dollars to build a new hospital on he premise for the care of the acutely ill.

I did not wait for all these changes. Now that my assignment was over, I decided to move on. When I told Fred that I had overstayed my job by two months and that I was planning set up a private practice at Cape Girardeau, he was rather upset. When he signed me up, he must have thought that I would continue to stay for years to come like most psychiatrists did in the past. But I reminded him that my original contract was only for one year and it was time for me to move on. I could see that Fred was not happy. Fanny Lou expressed a "sinking feeling" when she heard about my leaving. I was "manna from heaven" for the hospital, she said. The hospital staff gave me a sendoff party during which they gave me a deliberately dented trophy cup mounted on a marble pedestal. The inscription on it read: YOU'VE MADE SUCH A BIG DENT IN SO SHORT A TIME." A social worker came to me in tears and handed over a letter in which he expressed a great sense of loss. His letter summed up the sentiment of all staff members with whom I worked. I realized how a doctor leaving the hospital could be a great loss for the staff members. I am reproducing this poignant letter just to illustrate how one's sincere effort could affect others one encounters in life.

> *Bob,*
>
> *Sometimes I write better than I talk, so here it is in writing. And old American expression says, "You never miss your water 'til the well goes dry." Now that you're really leaving, I am just beginning to realize how much of a loss your departure will be. Though we were never close in many ways, we were still somehow close. I always felt a kinship and mutual respect, even when we were trying very hard to out talk each other. I will miss your warmth, support, and enthusiasm.*
>
> *My own loss seems relatively small when I think of the loss to the hospital. Where are we going to find a compulsive hypomanic who is bright, nice guy with charisma? Who the hell is going to provide leadership in the trenches? Who's going to charm the pants off the Medicare people? Who's going*

to teac the mew guys in Receiving Building what they didn't learn in school?

Please don't misunderstand —I don't think all those things are your personal responsibility. You just happen to have been doing that, shaping up the medical staff a bit, and then some.

Excuse (indulge?) my boring verbosity, please, for a few more lines. You cannot help but do well in your new practice. Whether or not I ever see you again, I will always consider you a friend. Even if what you might remember about me is giving you a hassle (and telling you I think you're full of crap), I wanted to be sure you also got the rest of my message.

Follow the path with heart.

R. H.

In 1987, the State of Missouri converted all the old buildings into a prison. In July 1987 a new building was inaugurated on the premise. I was not one of the invitees for this occasion, as none of the people involved in this project knew about my role in its creation. Southeast Missouri Mental Health Center at Farmington is now providing excellent care to patients from Southeast Missouri catchment area.

In On August 2, 1982, I opened my private practice in Cape Girardeau, Missouri, and never looked back. The psychiatric unit I started in Southeast Missouri Hospital in 1984 is still providing excellent care for seriously ill psychiatric patients. There were

numerous incidents all through my practice, which, if I recount here, would fill another 300 pages. The main lesson I learned from all these events was that there are no permanent friends; only permanent interests. Between 1982 and till my retirement on the Thanksgiving Day of 2010, I was privileged to have served thousands of wonderful people of this and surrounding cities. It was now time for me to begin the last phase of my life here on earth. I end this book by thanking them all for teaching me all that know about human nature and helping me to find myself.
THE END

Made in the USA
Charleston, SC
09 January 2017